150
WAYS TO BE A
SAVVY MEDICAL
CONSUMER

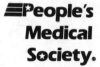
People's
Medical
Society.

OTHER BOOKS FROM
THE PEOPLE'S MEDICAL SOCIETY

150
WAYS TO BE A
SAVVY MEDICAL
CONSUMER

By Charles B. Inlander
President, People's Medical Society
and
The Staff of the
People's Medical Society

≡People's
Medical
Society.

Allentown, PA

The People's Medical Society is a nonprofit consumer health organization dedicated to the principles of better, more responsive, and less expensive medical care. Organized in 1983, the People's Medical Society puts previously unavailable medical information into the hands of consumers so that they can make informed decisions about their own health care.

Membership in the People's Medical Society is $15 a year and includes a subscription to the *People's Medical Society Newsletter.* For information, write to the People's Medical Society, 462 Walnut Street, Allentown, PA 18102, or call 215-770-1670.

This and other People's Medical Society publications are available for quantity purchase at discount. Contact the People's Medical Society for details.

© 1987, 1991, 1992 by the People's Medical Society
Printed in the United States of America

ISBN 0-9627334-5-8

CONTENTS

INTRODUCTION

It takes a savvy consumer to cut through the maze known as the American health care system. But with the right information, the right attitude, and a willingness to be just a little assertive, you can get quality health care at a cost far less than what many of your friends and neighbors pay.

Despite all its virtues, all its miracles, and all its victories, our health care system is fraught with physical and economic dangers. It is a system that even renowned medical experts have labeled "out of control."

There are 37 million Americans without health insurance. Another 30 million people are underinsured—they could not cover their medical bills if confronted with a major illness or a prolonged medical encounter. Corporations, which once provided liberal health care benefits to employees at little or no cost, now require employees to pay part of their insurance premiums, deductibles, and copayments. Some companies even have cut their benefits.

The numbers tell the story. In 1990 America spent 12.5 percent of the gross national product, or GNP, on health care. That's $660 billion, or more than twice what we spent on national defense. It also represented a 10.5 percent increase over the previous year. Overall inflation for the same period was 6.1 percent (and is falling).

But if those numbers don't hit home, try these. The average American household spends $6,750 each year for health care services. This includes out-of-pocket payments to doctors and hospitals, insurance premiums, medical equipment purchases, federal and state taxes used for health care, and the cost of health care benefits built into the goods and services you buy.

Under normal economic circumstances, health care costs should be going down. Demand is nowhere near the level of supply. Approximately 40 percent of the hospital beds in this country are empty. Every one of America's major cities has a doctor glut—many more doctors than we need in order to provide quality care to consumers. A coronary bypass procedure, which has increased in frequency by more than 100 percent in the last 10 years, went from an average of $20,000 per procedure in 1980 to $40,000 in 1990. Yet in the 1970s, when that particular operation was coming into vogue, medical gurus were promising a dramatic drop in cost as the operation became more commonplace. That's a pretty serious medical misdiagnosis.

Even the quality of American medicine is coming into question. Hospital infections are rampant. One out of 10 people who enter a hospital today can expect to acquire an infection they did not have when they were admitted. That is an almost 100 percent increase in the last decade. Twenty percent of all people who enter a hospital acquire a condition while in the hospital that they did not have before they came. Several studies have shown that up to 40 percent of the people admitted to hospitals are there as a result of something a doctor has done to them.

And while Americans get the most health care in the world, and pay the highest fees for it, overall the nation ranks relatively low, compared to other countries, in such categories as length of life and infant mortality.

As a result, consumers now are taking a more "buyer beware" attitude about medical services. We are questioning more, saying no to what appear to be useless or unnecessary services, seeking second opinions, using outpatient services, and entering wellness and rehabilitation programs.

The federal government, insurers, and businesses have implemented programs that require patients to get preapproval for treatments to ensure that the consumer is getting the right treatment for the condition presented. Medicare beneficiaries are staying fewer days in the hospital than before. Insurance companies are encouraging use of less costly outpatient services. Businesses are telling their employees to use fewer medical services and use them only when absolutely necessary.

Yet medical inflation continues to race ahead of the general inflation rate. What has happened is that instead of letting the normal laws of economics prevail, the benevolent and compassionate men and women who practice medicine, operate hospitals, manufacture medical equipment, and make drugs are raising their prices to make up for lost traffic. They have decided that they deserve a certain (and continually rising) level of income and profit, no matter how few customers they have.

But doctors and other medical and health care professionals usually deny they are business types. They talk about caring, healing, touching, and compassion. They tell us how hard and how long they work, the sacrifices they make, the terrible trials and tribulations of a life in the service of the sick and needy. But consumers have come to understand that beneath the white coat, behind the surgical mask, between the two tubes of the stethoscope resides a businessperson. And consumers are asking for the information and tools to deal with these professionals in a businesslike way.

That is why we wrote this book. Medicine is a business. While it is a business that deals with illness and the human condition, we must remember economics is always at play. Every time we use medical services, there is a cost attached. Unless we have insurance, we may not be "accepted" by a hospital or doctor. Doctors have signs in their offices asking people to pay at the time of visit. Hospitals post notices about minimum fees for use of the emergency room. No matter how helpful a medical service may be, the business element is always involved.

For the past several years, there has been a movement among business and government to contain the cost of medical care. The reality is that the cost-containment strategies employed by business and government have been successful in containing costs–but only for some businesses and the federal government. It has had very little effect on the average consumer, employee, or Medicare beneficiary. In fact, cost containment has not meant a reduction in fees, but rather a reduction in the amount of money spent by parties trying to contain their costs.

Twenty-seven years ago, when the Medicare program was launched, Americans over the age of 65 were spending 15 percent of their incomes for medical services. That predicament was the impetus for passage of the Medicare legislation. Citizens were outraged at these costs, and the Medicare program came into being. However, by 1990 something astounding had occurred. Medicare beneficiaries were now spending upwards of 20 percent of their incomes on medical care over and above what Medicare covered. In other words, the very economic conditions elderly people confronted in 1965 that brought about Medicare were even worse in 1991.

So much for the bad news. Now, what do we do as medical consumers? First, we arm ourselves with information–facts and figures that help us find the best care at the best price. Second, we formulate the questions that will get us the substantive answers we need from our health care providers.

And here's the good news. In the pages that follow, we have listed and explained 150 ways to be a savvy medical consumer. We have given you the facts and information that will help you find the best health care at the lowest price. Some of what you read, you may already know. Other ideas may never have dawned on you.

Every one of the 150 ways to find quality health care and lower your health care costs listed in this book works. They have worked for others just like you.

As president of the People's Medical Society, I am convinced that as individuals we can have quality health care and keep our personal expenditures down. As I travel around the country speaking to tens of thousands of people each year, they tell me what they have done to reduce costs for themselves. We have listed those methods in this book.

This book is your key for entering the world of quality health care and reasonable medical costs. We have tried to give you real actions you can take to make sure you receive the best medical care at the best price. (And believe me, I know they work. I have tried many myself.)

The staff of the People's Medical Society and I have reviewed all of these ideas. They are winners. And you too can be a winner over medical incompetence and medical inflation.

Read these ideas carefully. Use them at the next appropriate time. You will be surprised at just how easy it is to take charge of your own medical care. Do not be intimidated by medical professionals when you confront them. Remember, they are in business. And remember, so are you. It is your business to get the best care at the lowest cost.

This book will help you do that.

Charles B. Inlander
President
People's Medical Society

We have tried to use male and female pronouns in an egalitarian manner throughout this book. Any imbalance in usage has been in the interests of readability.

CHAPTER 1

Doctors

Doctors are the so-called gatekeepers of the medical world. Through them you enter the worlds of the hospital, laboratory, and pharmacy. But doctors are also much more. Not only do they determine the quantity of health care you receive and set the price, but they're also responsible for the *quality* of care you receive. Doctors control every aspect and avenue of the health care delivery system, and for these reasons–and more personal ones as well–you'll want to develop a good working relationship with your doctor. Knowing how to interact with a doctor makes you a smarter consumer, improving your prospects of getting high quality care. And by working carefully and assertively with your practitioners, you can greatly lower your health costs.

But first things first–how do you go about looking for Dr. Right? The fact of the matter is that most consumers spend more time selecting a roofer than they do choosing someone to look after their health. Choosing a doctor isn't easy. It's a process filled with questions, both for the prospective doctor and for yourself, but the savvy consumer will realize that the right choice will save money and perhaps even a life.

Begin your search by getting a few good recommendations from family members, friends, and neighbors. Word of mouth is still one of the best methods of finding out which doctors are taking new patients and what others think of these doctors. The old adage of "If you want to find a good doctor, ask a nurse" is probably a good one but not always practical. And don't overlook your present doctor, especially if your relationship with this doctor is ending because he is leaving practice or retiring. Ask him for names of other practitioners to consider. Other sources that may help you find a doctor are:

► *Doctor referral services operated by a local medical society (usually county-based).* Not necessarily our first choice, such services will refer only those doctors who are members of the society.

► *Hospital-sponsored physician referral services.* Similar to medical society referral services, in this case a local hospital refers you to a list of physicians who are either on their staff or have privileges at their facility. Neither referral service will comment on the specific ability of referred physicians other than to perhaps mention board credentials.

► *Newspaper advertisements of doctors announcing the opening of a new practice.* Be wary, however, and ask yourself why the doctor is advertising. To attract patients because she is just out of medical school? Or is in a highly competitive and glutted market? Or has she just moved in from a state where her license was revoked?

► *Your company personnel office.* Ask if your company maintains a list of doctors other employees have recommended.

► *Your health insurance company.* Check if your insurer has any local doctors to recommend or, in the area of a major problem, it recommends specialists for particular conditions.

► *Listings in the telephone directory.* Doctors' names are usually arranged according to practice or specialty, but be aware that just because a doctor says she specializes in a certain area of medicine does not mean the doctor actually took any advanced training in it. A doctor can practice in any specialty area she chooses.

► *Senior centers.* Some have referral services.

Here now are some savvy tips for dealing with doctors.

1.

Check for board certification.

Physicians who are board certified have to meet additional training requirements and must pass a rigorous examination administered by a specialty board. Since a large difference in fees between certified and noncertified physicians is unlikely, you may as well go with the doctor who has additional training–*if* he indeed does. Physicians know that consumers are more savvy about credentials, so they're doing everything they can to make themselves look better. So be alert to physicians who play a little game by putting initials after their name. They're counting on your being impressed when you see the initials "B.E." following their name. Don't be; it only means "board eligible."

Another favorite ploy of some physicians is to list themselves as board certified, but fail to tell you in which specialty. You've got to make sure that the physician is board certified in his main field of practice. To check the board-certification status of a physician, call the American Board of Medical Specialties. The group's toll-free number is 800-776-CERT. (When you call, have at hand the physician's full name and his city and state.)

2.

Ask for a get-acquainted visit.

Before seeking the professional services of a new doctor, we suggest that you contact several physicians to determine if they are accepting new patients. If they are, set up a short get-acquainted visit and offer to pay for the time. (According to a recent survey among physicians, the fee for a brief visit is between $22 and $35. Some physicians may not charge you for the time, but always offer to pay; it's one investment that will return dividends.) The purpose of this visit is to find out if you and the doctor see eye to eye on health issues and if her office services are efficient, and to have any of your questions answered *before* you commit to her services. No matter how thorough your doctor-shopping expedition has been, many problems do not arise until the first face-to-face encounter with the practitioner and the office staff.

3.
Check fees in advance.

There is a surprising amount of variation in basic fees, and, indeed, doctors tend not to publish or post their fees for a variety of reasons. The primary one is that they do not have a set fee for a given procedure. (The skeptic would say that the fees doctors charge have nothing to do with their qualifications—they are more likely to be due to the size of the doctor's mortgage or car payment.)

Each time you visit the doctor, ask what the charges will be for the procedures, tests, and treatments the doctor will perform. If the doctor does not know what his fees are, then insist that the person who does know come into the room with you and the doctor.

4.
Negotiate charges and fees.

Most people never think of negotiating with a doctor. Negotiating is something we do with a car dealer or a flea market vendor. The savvy consumer, however, never forgets that medicine is a business—in fact, the biggest business in America—and therefore, normal business practices apply, including negotiation.

Generally, doctors are willing to lower their standard fees for patients with limited incomes or special economic circumstances. Mind you, doctors probably won't readily admit that they negotiate their fees, but in reality they do. Every time a physician signs an insurance agreement, she is permitting someone else to set the price of service. Businesses have also taken actions that force employees to shop for the best price among physicians. By setting maximum reimbursement levels on insurance plans, businesses are telling employees to find the best value. Physicians are well aware of this practice and, because of increased competition, are more willing to adjust their fees in order to get the business.

Here's the strategy: If the quoted fee seems excessively high or is more than you can pay, tell the doctor. Indicate that you feel this is wrong or that you cannot afford such a cost. Ask if the fee can be lowered in your case or if some other payment scheme can be devised. If you have been using the physician for many years, call upon your loyal patronage. Remember, doctors' services are like airline fares: No two people are necessarily paying the same amount for the same class of service to the same destination. And just like the airlines, a doctor's financial security over the long haul is based on your repeat business.

5.

Make it clear to your doctor that all tests must be specifically approved by you before ordering.

Millions of medical tests are performed annually, and Americans and insurers spend billions of dollars for them. Yet many millions of these tests are not necessary, say some experts. And many of the tests aren't very accurate. Others have serious risks and iffy benefits. So you may well wonder—should you have that test? Does your malady really require two or three tests to determine a diagnosis?

The savvy consumer *can* take charge and *can* minimize the risks and costs of unnecessary or excessive testing.

▶ *Ask why you need the test.* Before you agree to any test, ask your doctor what will be done if the test results are abnormal and what will be done if the test results are normal.

▶ *Ask how reliable the test is, what the chance is of a false-positive or false-negative result, and how risks of either can be minimized.* (A false-positive result means that the test shows up positive, or abnormal, but no disease is actually present. A false-negative result means that the test shows up negative, or normal, but you actually have the disease.) Mind you, no test is 100 percent accurate, but you should be told the usefulness and the limits of tests if you are to make an informed decision.

▶ *Find out what alternatives you have if you refuse the test.*

▶ *Ask how much the test will cost.* And don't forget to check with your insurance company prior to undergoing an expensive test to see if it will cover the total cost.

6.
Check if the doctor uses an in-office laboratory.

In-office labs tend to be less expensive, but just as with any commercial laboratory, the test results are only as good as the people and equipment carrying out the test. Furthermore, regulations and standards governing in-office laboratories vary from state to state, and critics of office-based testing point to problems with accuracy, quality and quality control, lack of adequately trained laboratory staff and staff turnover–and incentive to profit through overtesting. Study after study shows small in-office laboratories tend to have a greater variability in test results than do large, regulated labs. Any one of these problems can take a toll on your health and finances.

So be sure to ask your doctor if her lab is inspected and certified. Find out the qualifications of the people working in the lab. What are their credentials? Is anyone a medical technologist, trained in the proper collection and preparation of specimens and the operation of the equipment? How often is the equipment inspected and calibrated, and when was the last time this was done?

7.
Discuss all options before agreeing to tests.

Doctors have come to rely on tests to such an extent that they tend to order them routinely, whether or not they're necessary to confirm a diagnosis. Discuss the necessity of each and every recommended test in detail with your doctor. Consult *The People's Book of Medical Tests,* by David S. Sobel, M.D., and Tom Ferguson, M.D. (New York: Summit Books, 1985) for more information on the test. Unnecessary medical testing, done solely as a defensive measure, costs consumers a whopping $15 billion a year!

Even in the area of testing, negotiation can play an important role. Let's assume the doctor recommends a particular test. Here's how to negotiate whether it is the most appropriate one for your current situation: Begin by asking why this particular test. Ask if there is a more comprehensive test that will answer more questions. Ask the doctor to explain the risks associated as well as matters like pain or time involved with the procedure.

Of course, ask the price and be prepared to pinpoint whether that price is all-inclusive.

When you get all the information, sit down with the doctor and negotiate what you want. Don't be afraid to ask more questions or make decisions that are not necessarily what the doctor might have originally recommended. Make sure this is a give-and-take situation. Ask the doctor, "If I do X, what are my chances that Y will occur?" In other words, come to an agreement.

In 1983 the People's Medical Society created the Code of Practice as a statement we believe each doctor should subscribe to. Ask your doctor to review it and tell you whether he or she will apply it to your care.

THE PEOPLE'S MEDICAL SOCIETY
CODE OF PRACTICE

I will assist you in finding information resources, support groups, and health care providers to help you maintain and improve your health. When you seek my care for specific problems, I will abide by the following Code of Practice:

I. Office Procedures

1. I will post or provide a printed schedule of my fees for office visits, procedures, tests, and surgery, and provide itemized bills.

2. I will provide certain hours each week when I will be available for nonemergency telephone consultation.

3. I will schedule appointments to allow the necessary time to see you with minimal waiting. I will promptly report test results to you and return phone calls.

4. I will allow and encourage you to bring a friend or relative into the examining room with you.

5. I will facilitate your getting your medical and hospital records, and will provide you with copies of your test results.

continued on next page

THE PEOPLE'S MEDICAL SOCIETY CODE OF PRACTICE
continued

II. Choice in Diagnosis and Treatment

1. I will let you know your prognosis, including whether your condition is terminal or will cause disability or pain, and will explain why I believe further diagnostic activity or treatment is necessary.

2. I will discuss with you diagnostic, treatment, and medication options for your particular problem (including the option of no treatment), and describe in understandable terms the risk of each alternative, the chances of success, the possibility of pain, the effect on your functioning, the number of visits each would entail, and the cost of each alternative.

3. I will describe my qualifications to perform the proposed diagnostic measures or treatments.

4. I will let you know of organizations, support groups, and medical and lay publications that can assist you in understanding, monitoring, and treating your problem.

5. I will not proceed until you are satisfied that you understand the benefits and risks of each alternative and I have your agreement on a particular course of action.

8.

Make it clear to your doctor that all consultations with other physicians must be specifically approved by you prior to ordering.

Especially during periods of hospitalization, you may find yourself being billed for consultations by specialists that you may not even have known took place, much less that you approved. Also check with your insurance company or employee benefits office before agreeing to any consultations; some companies require precertification, which means that the service, the consultation, or even the test must be approved in advance. Failure to get prior approval could reduce your benefit and result in a large out-of-pocket expense for you.

9.

Buy a medical guide to aid you in deciding whether or not to see a doctor.

There are several good home medical guides available that offer clear advice and instructions for determining whether a doctor's care is necessary. These are just a few such guides:

Mayo Clinic Family Health Book, edited by David E. Larson, M.D. (New York: William Morrow, 1990).

Take Care of Yourself: Your Personal Guide to Self-Care and Preventing Illness (4th ed.), Donald M. Vickery, M.D., and James F. Fries, M.D. (Reading, MA: Addison-Wesley, 1989).

The American Medical Association Family Medical Guide (rev. ed.), edited by Jeffrey R. M. Kuntz, M.D., and Asher J. Finkel, M.D. (New York: Random House, 1987).

The American Medical Association Home Medical Advisor, edited by Charles Clayman, M.D., et al. (New York: Random House, 1988).

The Columbia University College of Physicians and Surgeons Complete Home Medical Guide (rev. ed.), edited by Donald F. Tapley, M.D., et al. (New York: Crown, 1989).

The New Good Housekeeping Family Health and Medical Guide (New York: Hearst Books, 1989).

10.

Do not use a specialist as a primary-care physician.

A primary-care physician is one who cares for the whole patient and has not specialized in any one area of the body or condition. Adults have three types of primary-care physicians from which to choose:

▶ *General practitioners.* Though dwindling in numbers, some G.P.'s still practice today.

► *Family practitioners.* Doctors who intend to become F.P.'s take additional training beyond medical school—a three-year residency that covers certain aspects of internal medicine, gynecology, minor surgery, obstetrics, pediatrics, orthopedics, and preventive medicine—and then pass a comprehensive examination.

► *Internists.* Like family practitioners, these doctors complete a three-year residency and must pass a comprehensive examination, but they do not normally take training in pediatrics, orthopedics, and child delivery. Instead they have more advanced training in diagnosis and management of problems involving areas such as the gastrointestinal system, the heart, the kidney, the liver, and the endocrine system.

If you require the care of a specialist for a specific problem (such as a cardiologist for a heart problem), do not ask that person to treat any problems not related to that particular specialty. Not only are a specialist's time and care more expensive, but he may not be the best qualified to deal with problems outside of his specific area of expertise.

11.
Always go to a nonspecialist first— specialists are rarely necessary.

As you can see from the previous item, primary-care physicians are able to treat the vast majority of illnesses, and they will readily refer you to a specialist if necessary. But in the meantime you will have paid less for the care you received. Furthermore, self-referral to a specialist has potential problems. Sure, at some time or another any of us may need a specialist to help discover the cause of a troublesome problem or to manage an uncommon or uncomplicated disease; however, out of the obvious need for experts in fields of medicine has come an overspecialized, fragmented system of medical care. And out of this has sprung the phenomenon of, for example, the orthopedist who sees "the back problem" and not the person as a whole, the urologist who sees "the bladder infection" and not the person's complete medical condition, and so on. Specialization profoundly influences the way medicine is practiced. Too often patients are referred from doctor to doctor to be reassured that nothing is wrong with the organ system of the doctor's field of interest or specialty.

Self-refer only if you must and if you feel that you, alone or preferably with an advocate (a friend or relative) by your side, can maintain control over any decisions regarding tests, procedures, and so on. But first determine what type of specialist you need, or even if you need one. Furthermore, if you belong to a health maintenance organization (HMO) or preferred provider organization (PPO) and decide to see a specialist *first*–in short, self-refer, a practice that HMOs and PPOs frown upon–you could be responsible for the entire cost of the visit.

WHAT IS A SPECIALIST?

A specialist is a doctor who concentrates on a specific body system, age group, or disorder. After obtaining an M.D. (Doctor of Medicine) or D.O. (Doctor of Osteopathy) degree, a doctor then undergoes two to three years of supervised specialty training (called a *residency*). Many specialists also take one or more years of additional training (called a *fellowship*) in a specific area of their specialty (called a *subspecialty*).

How can you tell if a doctor is a trained specialist? A doctor who has taken extra training in his or her field often chooses to become board certified. In addition to the extra training, the doctor must pass a rigorous examination administered by a specialty board, a national board of professionals in that specialty field. A doctor who passes the board examination is given the status of *Diplomate*. Plus, most board-certified doctors become members of their medical specialty societies, and any doctor who meets the full requirements for membership is called a *Fellow* of the society and may use the designation. For instance, the title "FACOG" after a doctor's name denotes that he or she is a Fellow of the American College of Obstetricians and Gynecologists.

12.
Demand itemized bills.

Itemized bills are always a good idea because they let you know exactly what you are paying for and help you determine whether you are being billed for a service you did not receive. Sometimes even an itemized bill doesn't give you enough information to make such determinations. Hospitals and doctors use esoteric codes; if such codes appear on your statement, without explanation, contact the business office and ask for a statement in plain English. If you are still not clear about a charge, or have a dispute, ask your doctor to verify that a particular service, test, or product was ordered for your care.

13.
Use ambulatory care centers (or walk-in/walk-out centers) rather than hospital emergency rooms if your doctor is not available.

Anytime you feel you need a doctor's care, you should call your doctor first. But if your doctor is not available, an ambulatory care center (sometimes called urgicenter or emergicenter) is usually less expensive and less time-consuming than a hospital emergency room. Such facilities—either independent clinics or affiliated with hospitals—offer basic medical care on a walk-in basis for 12 or even 24 hours of the day, rather than only during traditional office hours. The mission in most primary/emergency/urgent care centers is to treat minor injuries or short-term illnesses and provide immediate treatment for routine problems: for example, cuts, sprains, dislocated or broken bones, sore throats, and earaches.

14.
Get a second opinion.

First isn't always best. It's odd, though—people are willing, even eager, to ask for seconds on just about everything, except medical diagnoses. It is always a good idea, for your health as well as your pocketbook, to get a second opinion on any invasive procedure your doctor recommends, whether diagnostic or surgical. Review the information on benefits in your insurance plan concerning when a second opinion is required and covered. Some companies require a second opinion for all elective procedures; however, if you forgo the second opinion, you may discover that your coverage has been reduced by half. But regardless of who pays, it is always smart to get a second opinion, especially if a trip to the hospital looms in your near future. Studies show that there is often substantial disagreement about diagnoses and treatment options.

15.
Get more than two opinions when the first two disagree.

If the second opinion does not agree with the first, it is often a good idea to get a third or even fourth opinion. What you are looking for is a consensus among practitioners, which allows you to make an informed decision about the best course of action. And thorough investigation on your part is the surest way to avoid unnecessary treatment and to save money in the long run.

16.
Get independent second opinions. Don't rely on a second opinion referral from your own doctor.

A lot of second opinion doctors recommended by first opinion doctors turn out to be professional ditto marks and not all that valuable in terms of independent judgments. This is true in part because surgeons are the doctors most often asked for second opinions, and they're hardly predisposed to recommend sheathing the knife. It's also true that doctors often refer patients to other doctors for nonmedical reasons, such as the fact that they're golf buddies or "I owe him a favor." You are less likely to get an impartial, objective second opinion from your doctor's friend or close colleague. In addition, chances are that your doctor will call and discuss your case with the person to whom he referred you, and the second opinion will be made before the second doctor has a chance to examine you.

To find your own physician for a second opinion, start by contacting your insurance company and requesting a list of physicians who participate in second opinion programs. Do the same with your employer's benefits manager and your union, if you're a union member. Check the *Directory of Medical Specialists* in your local library's reference section. Ask friends who might have had similar conditions what doctor they used. The point is—shop around to find the most objective and competent practitioner available.

17.

Explore the non-M.D. providers when possible.

Basic health care can often be provided competently, safely and less expensively by non-M.D.'s such as optometrists, podiatrists, chiropractors, audiologists, physician assistants, nurse-midwives, and nurse practitioners. A quick glance through the medical services section of the *Dictionary of Occupational Titles* will find hundreds of professional occupations concerned with treating and caring for sick and injured people. Some of these practitioners support and complement the services of doctors and dentists, while others practice independently, depending upon the laws of the particular state in which they are licensed.

These so-called limited license providers can save you money if used properly. As a savvy consumer, you should always check their credentials to make certain they are properly licensed or certified—especially important if your insurance plan requires that all non-M.D. providers must be licensed or certified in accordance with the laws of your state.

18.

Call ahead to see if the doctor is running on time.

Just as the savvy traveler calls the airport to see if a flight is on schedule, you can save a lot of time (and money, if you must take time off from work) if you call your doctor's office and ask whether appointments are running on schedule. And if you see a doctor regularly, ask the receptionist to call you if appointments are running late. This allows you to either adjust your schedule or change the appointment.

19.

Send the doctor a bill if she keeps you waiting for more than 30 minutes.

The idea that patients actually bill doctors for waiting time is no longer a novelty. (Not long ago a savvy Florida man sued his doctor for excessive waiting and won!) Medical practice management experts have taken note of this and are now telling doctors that they had better get used to it. One expert told a doctor to adjust the patient's bill for the next office visit. In short, value your time and remember that you have lost not only the time in the waiting room, but also the time it took you to get there and back.

20.

Use a doctor with separate waiting rooms for sick and well visits.

More and more doctors are offering this convenience, particularly for children. Doctors' offices are prime places to pick up illnesses, and more illnesses mean more money. How smart is it to pay to see a doctor, then pay again for something you "caught" in the waiting room? If your doctor doesn't provide such a service, recommend he do so.

21.

Make sure the doctor accepts your insurance coverage.

Always confirm, at the time you make the appointment, that the doctor accepts the health insurance that you carry *and* will accept your insurance reimbursement as "payment in full," less required copayments or deductibles. These three little words can lead to trouble if you and your doctor's billing staff are using the same words but speaking a different language. A simple misunderstanding here can lead to balance billing, the practice of billing the patient for the difference between the doctor's usual charge and the amount paid by the insurance company. Clarify these points ahead of time.

22.
Get a job in a hospital.

It may sound facetious, but it really can be a money saver. Hospitals often give employees free services—although in recent years some hospitals have modified their benefits plans to include deductibles.

23.
Make sure a family member becomes a doctor.

But don't pay for the relative's education!

24.
Don't offhandedly substitute an emergency room for your doctor.

Never go to an emergency room (except in absolute emergencies) unless you at least try to contact your doctor first. If your doctor does not make provisions for seeing people at relatively short notice during office hours, find another doctor. To avoid out-of-pocket expenses, check your insurance coverage concerning when ER visits are covered and when not. Another reason for avoiding the ER, if possible, is what you may encounter there. Less than desirable conditions and possibly a long wait. Some reports indicate that a wait of seven to 10 hours is not that unusual in certain cities and regions; so such a visit not only costs you more money, but it also wastes your valuable time.

If you are enrolled in a health maintenance organization (HMO), ideally your HMO will want you to use its emergency center or an affiliated hospital's emergency room for immediate treatment. However, as you know, not every emergency situation is so strategically and conveniently orchestrated. Find out your HMO's rules in the event you seek emergency care during night and weekend hours or away from home, as well as its rule should your calls to your primary-care physician go unanswered. Be smart and find out *ahead* of the time you *really* need this information.

25.
Seek telephone advice from your doctor whenever possible.

Most doctors are happy to answer questions and provide advice over the phone about medication, reactions to treatment, or recurring health problems. Ever since the People's Medical Society promoted the use of set-aside telephone hours in our physician Code of Practice (see pages 19 and 20), the concept has been catching on. You can save a considerable amount of money and perhaps unnecessary anguish by avoiding office visits for simple medical advice.

26.
Get to know your doctor's office staff.

Many problems can be solved and questions answered by a doctor's office staff, and, frankly, it's just smart to make yourself known to the people who control really important aspects of a medical practice. Patients are generally not charged for brief consultations with the office nurse – by phone or in person.

27.
Demand that the doctor accept Medicare payments on assignment.

Most doctors are willing to accept Medicare on assignment– which means that you will not be required to pay more than your 20 percent copayment–on a case-by-case basis. If your doctor is hesitant about accepting assignment, remind her that Medicare's new fee schedule will mean better and faster reimbursement. If your doctor refuses, find another doctor.

If you can't find another doctor, you can still save money on nonparticipating physicians (those docs who have not agreed to accept the Medicare-approved amounts as payments in full) thanks to limits on balance billing. New Medicare regulations limit the maximum payment to nonparticipating physicians, so they can't bill you for the full difference between the Medicare-approved amount and their regular fee if it exceeds 120 percent (in 1992) or 115 percent (in 1993).

28.
Read about your condition.

You will be able to make savvy, more informed decisions about your treatment–and avoid possibly unnecessary tests and procedures–if you know a lot about your condition and ask the logical and informed questions. Only then will you be able to be a major partner in making your health decisions. And don't neglect to take advantage of a free service right there in your own community: your local public library. If you have not discovered the resources, ingenuity, and helpfulness that a reference librarian has to offer, then by all means do so. Even if you live in a small community with a modest library, one with a limited catalog of medical and health books, there's always interlibrary loan. In addition, hospitals will often let you use their medical libraries.

29.
Say "No" if you do not understand, and ask questions until you do.

Never submit to a test, treatment, or procedure that you do not fully understand. You should be able to answer four questions about any treatment you doctor recommends:

1. What is the purpose of this test/procedure/medication?
2. How will it help my condition?

3. Are there less costly, and equally as safe, alternatives to what you propose?
4. What are the possible side effects, and what is the probability that one or more will occur?

Don't be intimidated by comments such as "Who's the doctor here?" or "It's to make you better." Every unnecessary test or procedure costs you money, not to mention time and possible discomfort.

30.
Demand a full justification of any tests or procedures.

Just as in number 29, you can make an informed decision about your doctor's recommendations only if you understand them and you know why a particular treatment is preferable to others.

31.
Look for free or low-priced community services.

Many communities offer flu shots, immunizations, simple screening tests, cholesterol screening, occult blood screening, and certain other health-related services through the county health department. Also visit health fairs in your area to learn more about services that are available in your community at no, or nominal, cost.

32.
Always ask if it is possible to use previous X rays rather than take new ones.

Doctors often order X rays because they do not know that previous X rays exist. Keep a complete record of X rays—what type, when, how many different exposures—and request that X rays be promptly sent to a new doctor. Even simple X rays are expensive (and can be dangerous), so they should be taken only if absolutely necessary.

33.

Avoid mobile X-ray units.

Mobile X-ray units often use miniature films that require a greater X-ray exposure. Also, these mobile units are used primarily for chest screening for tuberculosis, which is usually unnecessary.

34.

If you are a woman and under 50, consult your physician about the need for routine mammography.

In light of recent headlines on breast cancer rates, the savvy medical consumer who's a woman undoubtedly is wondering what to do and when. There is great debate among medical experts about when routine mammography is useful to begin. The benefits of mammography for women between the ages of 50 and 65 seem to be clear; studies done around the world show that regular screening mammograms can cut the death rate from breast cancer by 30 percent or more in these women. But among women between the ages of 40 and 49 or younger, the benefit of regular screening mammograms is much less clear, and the risk of undergoing unnecessary treatment (or not getting treatment you need) because of inaccurate results is much greater.

The American Cancer Society and the National Cancer Institute (along with nine other medical organizations, four of them professional radiology groups) endorse screening mammograms at one- or two-year intervals for women between the ages of 40 and 49. Two large professional groups, the American College of Surgeons and the American College of Physicians, have declined to recommend routine mammography screening for women 40 to 49 years old. And a panel of experts assembled by the U.S. Department of Health and Human Services recently concluded that mammography screening for women under 50 should be done only when there is a family history of the disease.

You should also remember that insurance companies usually will not reimburse for diagnostic tests that aren't medically necessary. This means that any such expense comes out of your pocket. In any case, be sure to discuss mammography thoroughly with your doctor.

35.

Avoid fluoroscopy if an ordinary X ray can do the job.

Fluoroscopy exposes you to much more X-ray radiation and, therefore, should never be used if a simple X ray will serve. Overkill on tests is a tendency many doctors have – and it's your wallet (and health) that suffers.

36.

Question routine preemployment X rays.

People whose jobs will require them to handle food or work with people are often required to be screened for tuberculosis by state laws. Nowadays there are perfectly acceptable non-X-ray tests to screen for tuberculosis that do not require radiation, so resist a chest X ray for this purpose.

37.

Refuse routine dental X rays.

Again, X-ray examinations are expensive and possibly dangerous, so you should never agree to them unless they are necessary to diagnose a problem.

38.

If you change dentists or go to a dental specialist, take your dental X rays with you.

There is no reason to submit to an additional set of X rays by a new dentist if you have had X rays fairly recently done. Just take your old ones along with you.

39.

Following three or more normal Pap smears one year apart, the Pap test may be performed less frequently at the discretion of your physician.

In 1988 the American Cancer Society adopted this policy, similar to that endorsed by the American College of Obstetricians and Gynecologists, the National Cancer Institute, and the American Medical Association. What's a good time interval? A recent study by researchers at the University of Washington in Seattle suggests that going more than two years without a Pap smear increases your risk of developing cervical cancer.

40.

Have routine screening tests done by non-M.D.'s.

In many cases routine screening tests can be done just as accurately by non-M.D.'s – for example, nurse-midwives in the case of Pap smears. It is usually more expensive to take the time of a fully qualified physician to perform simple tests than to use a nurse or other non-M.D.

CHAPTER 2

Drugs

You don't need to be an economist to know that the cost of prescription drugs has gone through the roof. In the 1980s inflation rose 58 percent, while in the same decade drug prices increased a whopping 152 percent. A prescription that cost $20 in 1980 now costs $53.76. And at that rate, it will cost $77.06 in 1995 and $120.88 in 2000.

What is a bitter pill for you, the consumer, to swallow is, on the other hand, a prescription for profit for the drug manufacturing industry. A 1991 report of the U.S. Senate Special Committee on Aging stated that while the average Fortune 500 industry in this country had an average profitability of 4.6 percent in 1990, the average profitability of the top 10 drug companies more than tripled that amount: 15.5 percent.

How can you stay on the winning side in this multibillion-dollar-a-year industry? Be savvy and protect yourself from the outrageous price increases. Think smart and know where to go to find out whether the drug your doctor prescribes for you is the best, most efficacious medication for your condition. Granted, in a nation that fills approximately 1.6 billion prescriptions each year and has some 2,500 drugs on the market, even the wisest of medical consumers cannot become familiar with the names of all the available prescription and over-the-counter medications. But the winning strategy is to arm yourself with information on as many "fronts" as you can: everything from choosing the best pharmacist and comparison-shopping for brand name, generic, and over-the-counter drugs to avoiding costly and potentially dangerous medication errors.

41.
Know your pharmacist.

A pharmacist can be an invaluable resource for information regarding drugs—any interactions to be aware of, alternative forms of the same drug (i.e., liquid or pills), and less expensive alternatives. You see, more than a pill counter, the pharmacist is the most readily accessible health care professional most of us have—a highly trained drug expert who probably knows more than your own physician about the relative benefits and risks of various drugs. With today's medications more complex and, in some cases, more potent, and with drug prescribing on the increase, the savvy medical consumer will find a competent and communicative pharmacist. It's also smart to talk with your pharmacist, for the better she knows you, the more she will be able to help.

WHAT A GOOD PHARMACIST DOES:
A CHECKLIST

✔ Does more than merely read a doctor's prescription, fill it, label it, and charge for it.

✔ Keeps important family medication records called patient medication profiles, and uses them to prevent allergic reactions to drugs, dangerous interactions, duplicate medications, and drug abuse.

✔ Advises how to use prescription and nonprescription medication; how and when to take it; what the possible side effects are; what the shelf life is; how to store the medication; and whether there is potential for dangerous interactions with foods and/or other medications.

✔ Answers your questions about the staggering variety of medicines, remedies, tonics, pills, elixirs, lotions, salves, capsules, and powders on the market.

✔ Advises you, when necessary, to seek a medical practitioner's help.

42.
Shop around for prescription prices.

Prescription drug prices vary about as much as a nervous stock market, and it's no secret that drug companies have raised their prices to wholesalers. So now, more than ever, you've got to become a determined shopper. On any given day you may be able to find better prices for the medications you need. Contact the large chain pharmacies first since they usually offer better discounts because of their bulk-buying practices. This, however, is not to say that a local pharmacy may not have a better price on a particular drug. Even if you have a prescription plan where you work, shopping for the lowest drug price is important, especially if you have a copayment based on a percentage of the total cost of the prescription.

43.
Buy generic prescription drugs whenever possible.

A generic drug (the name of which is usually a condensed version of the drug's original chemical name) is one whose active ingredients duplicate those of the brand name product. While a generic does not have to be the same size, shape, or color of the brand name, by law it does have to be bioequivalent, determined by how much of the drug is absorbed into the bloodstream and how quickly absorption takes place. A generic cannot differ from the pioneer drug by more than 20 percent in either the speed or amount of absorption.

So much for what it is, now why buy? On the average, generic drugs are 30 percent cheaper than their brand name cousins— even 50 to 70 percent cheaper than the more expensive medicines. Mind you, the generic is *usually* cheaper than the brand name drug, but always check with your doctor or pharmacist to determine whether a generic form of the drug you need is available, safe, and less expensive. Also, since laws vary across the country, ask what your state's law is concerning the substitution of generic for brand name drugs. The generic pharmaceutical industry can provide you with more information on generic drugs and their use. For a copy of their free guide, contact:

Generic Pharmaceutical Industry Association
200 Madison Avenue, Suite 2402
New York, NY 10016

10 OF THE MOST COMMONLY PRESCRIBED DRUGS AND THEIR GENERIC VERSIONS

Brand Name/Generic Name	Prescribed For
Amoxil/amoxicillin	antibiotic
Lanoxin/digoxin	heart
Zantac/ranitidine hydrochloride	ulcer
Premarin/conjugated estrogens	hormone
Xanax/alprazolam	anxiety
Dyazide/hydrochlorothiazide, triamterene	high blood pressure
Cardizem/diltiazem hydrochloride	heart
Tenormin/atenolol	heart
Naprosyn/naproxen	arthritis
Tagamet/cimetidine	ulcer

44.

Buy store-brand over-the-counter, or nonprescription, drugs whenever possible.

Many pharmacies and some grocery store chains purchase over-the-counter (OTC) drugs in bulk and package them under their own store's brand name or label. By reading labels you can compare prices on brand name items to the less expensive, but identical, store-brand item. But first, before you plunk down your cash for an OTC remedy with possibly questionable effectiveness, find out if a formerly prescription-only drug is available without a prescription. As the Food and Drug Administration (FDA) lifts the prescription-only restriction from many products, most notably decongestants and hydrocortisone, over-the-counter medications become available to treat the same symptoms that prescription drugs treat. The effectiveness of these medications has been proven, and it makes sense to spend your money for these products.

Indeed, Americans treat their ailments without professional help and often with nonprescription medicines some 60 percent of the time, according to an *American Pharmacy* article. Before you self-medicate, however, talk with your doctor or pharmacist about similar over-the-counter drugs. Remember, too, that some nonprescription drugs are as strong as the medications your doctor prescribes. As for the FDA's stamp of approval or the agency's eagerness to remove a suspect drug from the market, let's just say that ineffective and marginally effective drugs do exist.

A word of warning, though: The savvy medical consumer makes a point of consulting a pharmacist or physician before buying any OTC preparations for babies, young children, elderly or debilitated persons, or pregnant or breast-feeding women.

45.

Buy single-ingredient over-the-counter drugs.

Many over-the-counter drugs are preparations of several drugs, for example a "cold" medication that combines an antihistamine with a decongestant. It is less expensive to purchase a decongestant and an antihistamine separately—because often you will need only one of these to treat your symptoms and because mixtures can be more expensive.

Here are a few other wise strategies for selecting the best OTCs and getting the most for your money:

► Find out the risks or side effects of any OTC you're considering buying and taking.

► Ask about potentially dangerous interactions between over-the-counter medications and any prescription drugs you may be taking. Common products such as nose drops, antacids, and aspirin can interfere with the actions and effectiveness of prescription drugs.

► Go over with your pharmacist the label instructions of any medication so that you can be sure you're taking it wisely and appropriately—especially if you're taking drug preparations in forms you do not normally use or fully understand: suppositories or prolonged-release tablets, for instance.

46.
Break the code.

What we are talking about is shorthand code that doctors, pharmacists, and nurses share as part of a long tradition of cryptic communication that excludes consumers. Particularly prominent are the medical abbreviations that are scrawled across prescription forms. Fortunately for the smart medical consumer, translating those enigmatic terms into everyday language is not difficult. Here's a list of some Latin directions to pharmacists and common abbreviations that turn up frequently on prescription sheets (some doctors may use variations of these symbols):

Abbreviation (on prescription)	English meaning
ad lib.	as needed
a.c.	before meals
p.c.	after meals
b.i.d.	twice a day
t.i.d.	three times a day
q.i.d.	four times a day
h.s.	at bedtime
p.o.	orally (by mouth)
q.4h	every four hours
q.8h	every eight hours
ut dict.	as directed by doctor
OD	right eye (drops)
OS	left eye (drops)
OU	both eyes (drops)

47.
Ask for an initial one to two days' supply of any new prescription to check for side effects.

Since the possibility exists for an adverse reaction to *any* medication, you will save your health and money if you initially request only one to two days' supply of a new prescription. You can pick up the remainder of the prescription (and pay for it) the next day if no adverse reaction occurs.

48.

Ask your doctor for free samples.

Physicians regularly receive free samples of prescription and over-the-counter medications from pharmaceutical company representatives. Again, it's wise to initially stockpile only a few days' worth of an unknown drug until you are sure that you and it are compatible. Think of it as a test drive, something any savvy consumer would do first.

49.

Purchase drugs directly from your doctor.

Let us first say that the practice called physician dispensing is not without its critics; indeed, the entire issue has raised quite a hue and cry in the prescription drug industry lately—in part because it upsets the so-called natural order of business wherein doctors prescribe and pharmacists dispense. The pharmacists call it an encroachment on their territory and a source of potential harm to consumers. Meanwhile the doctors call it good for their patients and bottom-line smart for their incomes.

What has made this a growth industry is a relatively new business called "repackaging": Companies (called repackagers) buy drugs in bulk at wholesale costs from drug manufacturers, then resell to doctors in convenient, safety-sealed containers, ready for on-the-spot dispensing to their patients.

Frankly, the answer to the question "Is physician dispensing a patient convenience or exploitation?" has more to do with the individual physician than with the practice as a whole. So the savvy medical consumer will get all the facts before buying and taking any prescription drug dispensed by her physician:

▶ Compare the doctor's prices with those of area drugstores to determine whether there is an economic advantage to the consumer.

▶ Verify if anyone in the doctor's office assures that the drugs dispensed are the right ones, the dosages correct, and the directions clear, complete, and accurate. (After all, physician dispensing sidesteps the highly trained drug expert, the pharmacist.)

50.
Purchase in bulk, when appropriate.

Although individuals cannot buy drugs directly from wholesalers, bulk purchasing is a way you can purchase your medications in larger quantities. If you're taking a certain medication for an extended period of time, have your physician write the prescription for a six-month or longer supply, as opposed to six refills. Some pharmacists may be wary if you ask for your six refills all at once, and your state's pharmacy laws may prohibit such dispensing. That's why it's better to have your physician write in the number of pills–such as 200 or 250–then you can discuss bulk purchases with the pharmacist.

51.
Investigate purchasing by mail order.

The cost savings of doing such, according to the industry's trade organization, range anywhere from 5 to 40 percent off prices at your local pharmacy. The American Association of Retired Persons offers a full-service mail-order pharmacy to members, a program that generally has lower prices than regular pharmacies. Other mail-order businesses offer more specialized medications such as homeopathic remedies and vitamin and mineral supplements. Just make sure that prices are indeed lower before purchasing by mail.

52.
Ask about any available discount.

Many, if not most, pharmacies offer senior citizen discounts. Infants' and children's discounts are also available in some pharmacies. Ask the pharmacist for details.

53.

Purchase a prescription plan.

Most group health insurance policies offer prescription coverage for a small additional premium. Ask if your plan offers this additional coverage as an option.

54.

Keep a patient medication profile on yourself (or make sure someone else is doing so).

No doubt about it—someone should be keeping a medication profile on you, indeed on everyone in your household. It's a system that monitors all the drugs you are taking, in hopes of avoiding medication errors. Actually, the logical site for the profile is your pharmacy. The American Pharmaceutical Association recommends that a patient medication profile contain the following information:

▶ Your name, address, and phone number.

▶ Your and your family's birthdays, so that the pharmacist can check whether the dosage is appropriate to the age of the user.

▶ Any allergies, reactions, or adverse effects you've demonstrated.

▶ A concise health history, including any conditions or diseases that would preclude the use of certain drugs.

▶ The over-the-counter, or nonprescription, medicines you take.

▶ The date and number of each prescription filled for you, the name of the drug, its dosage and strength, quantity, directions for use, and price.

▶ The prescriber and dispenser of every medication you take.

55.

Properly store drugs.

Most drug items need to be kept fresh, just as many food products do, with cool, dry conditions best for preserving them. True, some people, especially those who might in an emergency need to get to their medications at a moment's notice, like to keep multiple vials of their prescription drugs stashed away–in the kitchen, in the bedroom, in the workshop, or even in the car. But tossing pills in with the maps and owner's manual is a prescription for trouble–and meltdown. Ask your pharmacist how to store the drugs you are purchasing.

56.
Guard against overmedication.

It's a fact that drug overdosing occurs in many hospitals' pediatric wards and nurseries. The dosages–some as much as 10 times greater than prescribed–are the result of misplaced decimal points and sloppy computational skills of nurses and doctors who do not understand the appropriate doses for different age groups. But that's not all. Various reports have pointed out that drug overdosing occurs with the low-weight elderly. Not only are doctors failing to adjust doses for body weight in many cases, but they often also do not take into account the ages of the patients. The operative physiologic fact here is that the older you get, the longer it takes for drugs to clear out of your system, so dosages must be adjusted accordingly.

It just makes sense, doesn't it, that correct dosages vary among people just as their ages and weights vary? If a savvy medical consumer knows this, shouldn't a doctor? Well, the problem, according to one study, is that doctors prescribe "by habit, with little adjustment for individual patients." So the next time your doctor writes a prescription for you, ask her to double-check your weight and age against the recommended standard dosage for that medication. It may mean a double-savvy whammy: You'll save money if the effective drug dose is less, and you'll increase your margin of safety for dose-related side effects.

57.
Purchase drugs from your HMO pharmacy.

If you are a member of a health maintenance organization (HMO), find out if it has an in-house pharmacy. HMO pharmacies often sell drugs to members at wholesale cost or slightly above.

58.

Consult drug reference books.

To learn more about the medications that are prescribed for you and your family, consult a drug reference guide. You'll find them in libraries as well as pharmacies. A good guide will list the medication by class—such as an antidiabetic or a calcium channel blocker—by chemical or generic name, and by brand name. There should also be a section in which the medication is described and the condition(s) given for which the medication may be prescribed. Additional sections usually discuss how to use the medication; when not to use it in conjunction with other medications; and what the side effects and contraindications (reasons you shouldn't use the medication) are.

Two good reference guides are the *Physician's Desk Reference* and *The Complete Drug Reference,* the latter published by Consumer Reports Books. A reference librarian can help you locate other sources of prescription drug information. Clearly, the best time to find out that a drug may not be appropriate for you is before you have gone to the expense of having the prescription filled.

59.

Consult consumer buying guides to drugs.

Buying guides to drugs, written especially for consumers, are available in most libraries. In addition to giving you information about specific medications, they also point out which drugs are the most effective and which drugs are not effective. Using the most effective drug for a given condition is ultimately cheaper. Some guides you may want to look for are:

Fifty Plus: The Graedons' People's Pharmacy for Older Adults, Joe and Teresa Graedon (New York: Bantam Books, 1988).

The New People's Pharmacy Book: Drug Breakthroughs for the 1980s, Joe Graedon (New York: Bantam Books, 1985).

Worst Pills, Best Pills, Sidney Wolfe, M.D., et al., (Washington, DC: Public Citizen Health Research Group, 1988).

CHAPTER 3

Hospitals

Where you get your medical care is as important as who provides it. The backdrop not only dictates what treatment you get or do not get, but it makes a *big* difference in how much you pay.

You don't have to be a cost accountant to realize that certain health care settings are more expensive than others, with hospital-based care the steepest. One night in a hospital costs an average of $297 or a total of $2,138 for an average stay (December 1991 figures). And that covers only the room and meals; when drugs, medical tests, and other charges are factored in, the daily cost climbs sharply to $900. In terms of national impact, the dollars and cents quickly add up. In 1991, $256 billion was spent for hospital care. That amounts to $1,024 for every man, woman, and child in the country.

Dollar figures like these are enough to convince most people to reduce the time spent in the hospital, if not completely eliminate hospitalization in favor of another setting. But if you must go in, pay close attention to procedures and medications ordered by your physician, and make sure you know what has been ordered and that you are fully informed of the whys and wherefores. Further, if you must go in, it stands to reason that a close scrutiny of the entire process, from preadmission talks with your doctor, to admission, and on to discharge, has the potential to save you money *and* gets you intimately involved in important decisions about your health and welfare.

Speak up whenever you find something is not what you have been told. Be on the lookout for errors in medications, procedures, and the like that can end up costing you extra days in the hospital, as well as extra money from your pocket.

Using even one of the following money-saving hints will save you *at least* the price of this book. And that's just savvy personal finance!

60.
Don't go unless absolutely necessary.

An unnecessary stay threatens far more than your wallet, as if money alone weren't enough to quibble over the necessity of hospitalization. Hospitals can be hazardous to your health. While in the hospital you are at risk of piling up mounds of charges for procedures and tests, but you are also at risk of acquiring a condition you did not have when you went in. That happens to one out of every five hospital patients, and these conditions not only require additional treatment at additional cost, but they can be deadly as well. One of these so-called iatrogenic (literally, doctor-produced) conditions—nosocomial infection—is produced by microorganisms that dwell with relative impunity in hospitals. Most develop at least 72 hours after admission, which means that some may not become manifest until after discharge.

You could describe nosocomial infections as expensive souvenirs of your hospital stay. And close to one out of every 10 patients admitted to a hospital acquires one of these nasty, and often preventable, souvenirs. It is estimated that the recovery time necessary to combat a nosocomial infection is about four extra days of stay. Expensive as it is—experts estimate that it adds, at a minimum, $2.5 billion to America's medical bill—nosocomial infections can also be deadly souvenirs: Some tallies of infection-related deaths run as high as 100,000 (other estimates are even higher, 300,000 or so) a year.

What does the savvy medical consumer do, however, who needs a particular medical procedure? If you require a surgical procedure, you may be able to avoid the hospital entirely if the surgery can be done on an outpatient basis—you're in by around

9 a.m. and out by 5 p.m. or so. Ask your physician about this option. Outpatient surgery is usually less expensive than inpatient surgery, and you lessen the risk of picking up a nasty germ while in the hospital. In fact, your insurance plan or your employer may require you to investigate outpatient surgery first.

There's also the matter of copayment, that cost-sharing requirement in many insurance policies in which you assume a portion or percentage of the cost of covered services. If your copayment is 20 percent on inpatient services and only 10 percent on outpatient services–a not unlikely scenario–it's to your advantage to select the outpatient setting.

61.

Make sure hospital personnel wash their hands before touching you.

Of all the potentially protective measures you can take (or insist that your caregivers take), this one merits its own individual mention. Why? Well, because most of the hospital-acquired infections are gotten from the contaminated hands of doctors, nurses, and other hospital personnel. The Institute for Child Health Policy and others report that many hospital workers who come in direct contact with patients don't take the time, or are not concerned enough, to perform the simplest and best known of precautionary actions. And doctors are among the worst offenders. You can greatly lower your chances of catching such an infection–and paying for its treatment–simply by refusing to allow hospital personnel to care for you until they have washed their hands.

62.

Protect yourself from nosocomial infections.

There is no surefire defense for you if the rest of the hospital is a vast and bubbling breeding ground. So the first step is to try to gain admission to a hospital that has a good nosocomial record. Ask your doctor about it. Contact your local department of health. Ask the hospital directly, but be on your guard if the hospital paints too rosy a picture. That may mean that the staff is not properly surveying the facility's infection rate, or not surveying at all.

The other line of defense is to be informed. Remember, a savvy medical consumer is armed with information. Know the work areas of the hospital where you are at higher risk:

▶ *Hemodialysis unit.* The equipment here can be a source of hepatitis B, a virulent organism that is difficult to destroy.

▶ *Intensive care unit.* Usually occupied by patients who are extremely weak and thus susceptible to infection, this unit is operated under emergency measures that often have to forsake pristine sanitary procedures in order to save a life.

▶ *Infant nursery.*

▶ *Operating room.*

Nosocomial infections can also pass to patients via the procedural chain of the food services department, due to any one or more factors – nearly all of them with their roots in human error. And a myriad of studies also point to other work areas in the hospital that, because of persistently poor and unprofessional hygiene practices, are breeding grounds, too: the central service department (the unit responsible for processing, storing, and dispensing hospital supplies); the pharmacy; the laundry; the laboratory (where, more than one story goes, workers have to be admonished not to keep their lunches in the same refrigerators as the ones that contain serum or other specimens).

63.

Assert yourself.

While it is true that one-third of all infections treated in hospitals are nosocomial infections, it is also estimated that as many as half are preventable. The savvy medical consumer is, where necessary, assertive. Here are some actions you can take while in the hospital:

▶ If your roommate becomes infected, or if you are concerned that what he or she has could possibly be transmitted to you via the air or through the use of a common bathroom, ask your doctor or the staff nurse-epidemiologist about your risks. Change your room at once if there is any chance you might become infected, because once you are infected it is too late.

► If you are undergoing surgery or a procedure that requires the removal of hair, refuse to be shaven the night before surgery. One study indicates that among people shaved the day prior to their operations, the nosocomial infection rate is 5.6 percent. Chemical depilatories reduce the rate to just 0.6 percent. Using barber clippers to remove hair the morning of surgery yields a low infection rate, too.

► Question whether shaving or clipping is necessary at all. Maybe not—and especially when it comes to ob-gyn situations. Removing hair before vaginal delivery or surgery in that area is probably uncalled for, because the old idea that hair creates a climate for infection is unsubstantiated by clinical studies.

► Have nurses regularly check the drainage of urinary catheters to help maintain cleanliness.

64.

If you deliver your baby in the hospital, get him or her out of there as soon as possible.

Although this advice is somewhat tongue-in-cheek, there is a valid reason for concern. Birthing in hospitals exposes infants to the full range of hospital-acquired infections to which adults are exposed. Upper-respiratory and "staph" infections are common in hospital nurseries. And, aside from the worry you will expend, you are required to pay for the care required to treat these infections.

65.

Refuse admission tests that are not pertinent to your illness or the reason for your hospitalization.

Most hospitals routinely require a variety of blood and urine tests and an X ray upon admission, whatever your age and physical health and whether or not you need them. The American College of Radiology has urged that chest X rays be eliminated as a routine procedure for hospital admissions, tuberculosis screening, and preemployment physicals, and as a general rule it's good to avoid X rays unless absolutely necessary because of the dangers associated with excessive radiation. It is in the best interest of your physical and financial health to refuse unnecessary routine testing.

66.
Use outpatient services.

Many invasive diagnostic tests and simple surgeries can be done on an outpatient basis, an arrangement whereby you arrive in the morning for the procedure and are back home again in the afternoon or evening. As an outpatient you are not officially admitted as an inpatient to the hospital, but you receive hospital care (for example, laboratory work and X rays) without occupying a hospital bed or without receiving room, board, or general nursing care. The growth in outpatient care has been so phenomenal that more and more insurance companies are requiring that certain procedures be done on an outpatient basis—mainly because of the cost savings associated with that setting versus inpatient care. Make sure that you know the requirements and limitations of your insurance coverage; otherwise you may end up paying substantial out-of-pocket costs. Remember, the less time you spend in the hospital, generally the cheaper it will be—and as we discussed before, the less likely you are to acquire a nosocomial infection.

67.
Don't stay overnight for diagnostic tests.

Most diagnostic tests can be done on an outpatient basis, in and out in one day. Again, if you don't have to spend a night in the hospital, don't do it. Remember, any stay in a hospital entails money *and* potential exposure to unwanted illness.

68.

Go to the hospital that does the largest number of the procedure that you need.

Studies have shown that you are less likely to suffer complications or die if you have your surgery or other invasive procedure done at a hospital that performs a large number (some experts recommend at least 200 per year) of such procedures. You save yourself a lot of money and untold amounts of suffering if you do what you can to assure the best outcome from the start. After all, you pay the price in more than dollars for their mistakes or inadequacies.

69.

Avoid for-profit hospitals.

Along with the family farm, the independent community hospital is fast becoming a lone ranger. Hand in hand with the burgeoning for-profit hospital business has come a rise and monumental growth in corporate chain ownership. Today the top three for-profit medical corporations—Hospital Corporation of America, Humana, and American Medical International—either own or manage nearly 87,000 beds in 530 hospitals nationwide. Current estimates are that for-profit hospitals tend to be more expensive—as much as 23 percent more expensive. Recently, a particular for-profit hospital chain was found to have marked up supplies anywhere from a few hundred percent to 4,000 percent. Such economics may explain why a $3 pill costs up to $29 in one of these for-profit facilities. And who pays for this markup? You, your employer, and your insurance company all pay for these outrageous charges.

The savvy medical consumer's strategy is this: Before your doctor arranges for you to be admitted to a certain hospital (assuming, of course, that your condition does not require emergency care), find out who owns it and how that ownership might affect your care and its cost. Call the hospital and ask for the hospital administrator's office. Ask the administrator who owns the hospital. Ask if it is nonprofit, owned by a religious order, or part of a large conglomerate that owns many more facilities around the country. Know the setup before you become a patient.

70.
Check room rates in advance.

There are differences in room rates from hospital to hospital. The basic charge for a hospital room may vary from $250 to $500 a day depending upon the type of hospital and region of the country. The cost of ancillary services (lab, supplies, nursing, etc.) can easily add an extra $500 a day. If you have an insurance plan that pays only up to a certain amount, say $350 a day, you've got to shop around for an affordable room.

71.
Refuse to pay a hospital admitting fee or hospital release (or discharge) fee to your doctor.

These fees, which are commonly charged by doctors for admitting and discharging you from the hospital, are unjustifiable on the basis of services rendered to you, the patient. Find out whether your doctor customarily charges such fees and discuss your objections prior to your admission to the hospital.

72.
Negotiate a discounted fee with your doctor in exchange for allowing services of a resident.

If you have no objection to having your surgery or other procedures performed by a resident physician, then make that clear to your doctor. Just remember that is how residents learn. But make sure that you do not pay for more than you get.

73.
Avoid cesarean-section deliveries.

A recent study showed that more cesarean sections are performed at night and on weekends– partly because doctors want to get the delivery over with quickly and therefore are less willing to wait through a long labor.

Cesarean-section deliveries are major surgery. They are not only much more expensive than vaginal deliveries, but they also expose both mother and baby to additional risks. Further, studies show that only one out of four women who had a previous cesarean-section delivery need have another one for the birth of subsequent children. The adage of "Once a cesarean, always a cesarean" is just not true. Indeed, the American College of Obstetricians and Gynecologists issued strong guidelines some years back stating that repeat cesarean deliveries should no longer be routine.

The best way to avoid a cesarean-section delivery is to be as knowledgeable as you can about the birth process so that you will be better able to ask the right questions and evaluate your doctor's recommendations. Not all cesareans are avoidable, but a good many are–and with information on whys, wherefores, and options you can avoid being one of those.

74.
Use a nurse-midwife or family practitioner as your birth attendant and consider alternative birth settings.

At the outset let us say that, clearly, where birth attendants and settings are concerned, different strokes for different folks. The savvy–and pregnant–medical consumer realizes that the type of childbirth experience she has depends very much on who she finds to deliver her baby and where she decides to have it.

There are two reasons you save money by choosing a practitioner other than an obstetrician as your birth attendant: Other birth attendants usually charge less in basic delivery fees, and they generally will not recommend a costly cesarean section or other expensive (and potentially dangerous), high-technology interventions unless they are absolutely necessary. For more information on nurse-midwife services, contact:

> American College of Nurse-Midwives
> 1522 K Street, N.W., Suite 1000
> Washington, DC 20005
> 202-289-0171

Developed by midwives believing it to be the best alternative to both hospital and home deliveries, the birth center ideally offers a home*like* environment, a relaxed, flexible atmosphere, and very little intervention in the birth process. Birth centers are designed to provide maternity care to women judged to be at low risk of obstetric complications, and this approach enjoys a loyal following of doctors, midwives, childbirth educators, and consumers who champion the low complication and cesarean-section rates, safety, consumer satisfaction, and cost savings that many birth centers offer. A 1989 survey showed that, for normal birth, birth centers offer a 35 to 47 percent cost savings over hospitals, depending on the length of stay. For more information, contact:

> National Association of Childbearing Centers
> 3123 Gottschall Road
> Perkiomenville, PA 18074
> 215-234-8068

There is also growing interest in home births, and if your insurance plan will cover such services it's worthwhile to investigate your options. For more information, contact:

> National Association of Parents and Professionals for
>   Safe Alternatives in Childbirth
> Route 1, Box 646
> Marble Hill, MO 63764
> 314-238-2010

75.

Become acquainted with the hospital's birthing policies and routine services before choosing to deliver there.

From a cost perspective, you should be looking for hospital policies that encourage "rooming-in" (keeping the baby in the room with you) and early discharge (generally after 24 hours rather than three days). Often hospitals charge for routine birth services—such as enemas, IVs, and use of the delivery room—that not every woman has. Scrutinize the bill and don't pay for any service you didn't receive. (And don't permit your insurance company to either.) By the way, the average charge for a hospital-based birth is $4,300 ($7,200 for a cesarean section).

76.

Do not routinely circumcise your male babies.

Circumcision is an operative procedure for which hospitals charge around $75. It is recognized to be unnecessary for health reasons; consequently, more and more health insurance companies are refusing to pay for this procedure. For more information, contact:

> National Organization of Circumcision Information
>   Resource Centers
> P. O. Box 2512
> San Anselmo, CA 94979-2512

77.

Demand itemized bills.

Ongoing studies by national hospital bill auditing firms consistently show that upwards of 90 percent of all hospital bills contain errors—miscalculations that are seldom in your, the consumer's, favor. In fact, the situation has gotten so out of hand that businesses are now offering "bounties" to employees who can spot the inaccuracies in their bills. The reward is a split of the money recovered from the hospital.

The problem here is that you can spot these errors only if you receive an itemized bill, which in most cases will not be given to you unless you ask for it. Scrutinize the bill closely, looking for any supplies, services, procedures, tests, or whatever that you did not receive.

If your bill is going to be paid by your insurer, be sure to inform your insurer directly, and in writing, of any inaccuracies in the bill. Everyone saves money by making sure that insurers do not overpay hospitals.

HOSPITAL BILLING ERRORS: WHAT TO LOOK FOR

American Claims Evaluation, Inc., another firm in the business of auditing hospital bills, recommends that you ask yourself the following questions to help identify possible errors on a bill. Clearly, these do not cover every possible misbilling, but they are a good start:

1. Was I billed for the right kind of room (semiprivate, private, etc.)?
2. Was I billed for the correct number of days I occupied the hospital room?
3. Was I billed correctly for any time spent in specialized units (intensive care unit, coronary care unit, etc.)?
4. If I left before "checkout time," was I billed for an extra day even though I'd already gone?
5. Was I billed only for those X rays and tests that I actually received?
6. If I had preadmission testing, did the hospital bill me for the "standard admission test battery" even though I never had it?
7. Was I charged only for supplies, medications, therapy, dressings, injections, etc., that I received? Were the quantities correct?
8. Were medications that my doctor prescribed billed over the entire stay even though I took them only once or twice?
9. Were drugs prescribed for me to take home actually received?
10. Was I billed for bedpans, humidifiers, admission kits, thermometers, etc., that I never received and/or was not allowed to take home?

78.

Keep a diary to compare with the hospital bill.

Document all medications, tests, and procedures, and compare your list with the itemized hospital bill. Make sure that individual items match those you actually received, and that you are not billed for more items than you received. Again, if you didn't use or undergo it, don't pay for it. You'll find a complete hospital diary in the back of the People's Medical Society book *Take This Book To The Hospital With You* (New York: Pantheon, 1991), along with a hospital evaluation form that should be sent to the People's Medical Society.

79.

Make sure you get what you pay for.

Many hospitals are teaching hospitals, which means they have a staff of medical interns and residents who work with "attending" physicians (such as your doctor). Unfortunately, this means that although you are paying full fees to your doctor, he may be doing very little of the work. You should specify, in writing, that any surgery or invasive procedure be done by the person you are paying for the service. If you are paying for a fully-trained physician, that is who you should get.

80.

Refuse to be seen by any doctor you don't know.

If any doctor you do not know enters your hospital room to see you, you can be sure you will receive a bill for his "services" (often nothing more than a quick glance into your room) unless you immediately make it clear that you do not want those services. Find out who these doctors are and why they are there, and make sure you or your insurer does not pay later for the services.

81.

Have a friend or relative with you to act as advocate.

As a hospital patient, it is very difficult to be an assertive consumer. Always bring along a friend or family member to act as an advocate, whose most important task will be to make sure you do not agree to anything without fully understanding it. In many cases, these personal advocates may have to stay with you 24 hours a day.

Many hospitals have on staff a so-called patient advocate, who supposedly can help you resolve minor problems. While we can't vouch for the effectiveness of every patient advocate, it's a good idea to at least become acquainted with this person. Let this person know that you're an informed consumer and won't hesitate to call upon him if a situation should arise. And don't forget to bring to the hospital your copy of *Take This Book To The Hospital With You,* the People's Medical Society's guide to surviving your hospital stay.

82.

Die at home.

Over 50 percent of medical costs are incurred in the last five days of life. Of course, the decision about where to die is very personal and one that many never get the opportunity to make. But it is a valid consideration—for many reasons, including cost—and should be given serious thought.

83.

Make a living will.

A living will is a legal document that is used to inform family and medical personnel of your wishes concerning medical care, should you be unable to personally make those wishes known. These documents are most often used to limit the types of medical care you wish to receive if you are known to be in a terminal stage of illness. For instance, a living will may proscribe the use of an artificial life-sustaining treatment, such as an automatic ventilator.

As of 1992 every hospital is required by law to ask you if you have a living will or any other type of directive that can be followed if the issue should arise. The law does not require you to have such directives nor does it mean you must make one up. It merely requires hospitals to ask.

There are many reasons, in addition to the cost considerations, to choose to have a living will. No matter what your reasons, it is a good idea to discuss your living will with both your family and your doctor. And prepare your family to fight for your right to the choices expressed in the living will should you personally be unable to do so.

If you do have a living will, make sure you give a copy to your family doctor and any other physician you regularly use. If you are brought to a hospital unconscious or with no family member present, contact may be made with one of these doctors, who can then pass along your instructions.

To obtain more information on living wills and durable power of attorney for health care—the latter, another form of advance directive—contact:

> Choice in Dying, Inc.
> 250 West 57th Street
> New York, NY 10107
> 212-246-6973

84.

Bring your own food.

Hospital meals are expensive (and, frankly, not always edible), partly because of the costs of hiring clinical dietitians who order menus based upon patients' nutritional needs. But if you are permitted to eat a normal diet, you will not need any special food and can save a lot of money—and keep your taste buds happy in the process—by providing your own food. (Skeptics of hospital food—and there are many, including probably most people who have ever eaten such food—maintain that you won't miss much either.) This strategy may also be necessary if you are on a restricted, such as vegetarian or kosher, diet. Remember, though, that providing three meals per day is hospital routine. So make it explicit that you do not want the meals and will not pay for them.

85.
Bring your own drugs.

This is a savvy (and easy) money-saving technique. Bring to the hospital an adequate supply of any medications you take (making sure beforehand, of course, that your doctor is aware of your usual medication regimen and has documented such in your hospital record). Medicate yourself at the appropriate times. It is also a good idea to take along some basic analgesics such as aspirin or acetaminophen, if you use them. Hospitals charge a lot ($3 for two aspirin tablets, in some cases) for medications.

If you are unable to medicate yourself, ask a family member to help. Have your doctor inform the nurses of such an arrangement.

86.
Bring your own vitamins to the hospital.

Hospitals do not ordinarily supply vitamin or mineral supplements–and if they did, you can be sure it would be at an exorbitant price. So if you customarily follow a vitamin and mineral supplementation regimen, bring them with you. And make sure the doctor marks on your chart that you are to be given your own vitamins, or that supplements are to stay in your possession so you can take them yourself.

87.
Avoid weekend admission.

Don't allow yourself to be admitted on a nonemergency basis on a Friday afternoon or evening. You will just languish, expensively and in no particular comfort, until Monday. Most of the labs that would be performing your diagnostic workups don't do those things on weekends. Weekend admission equals one to two days extra in the hospital, at your expense. Only basic care is performed on the weekend. Wait until Monday; better yet, Tuesday, some experts say. By Tuesday the hospital is back in gear after the weekend and the end-of-the-week blahs haven't hit yet.

88.

Complain if you are being disturbed.

Hospital personnel are accustomed to dealing with uncomplaining, often drugged patients. If your room is noisy at night or your sleep is disturbed, complain. A *British Medical Journal* report some years back cited more than 20 studies that responded resoundingly yes to the question "Is sound, prolonged sleep essential for optimal healing?" The savvy medical consumer will make sure that adequate rest periods of uninterrupted sleep are part of the care plan.

CHAPTER 4

Laboratories

Over- and unnecessary testing and errors in test results are problems you've got to be on the lookout for. They can do irreparable harm to your pocketbook—*and your health*, if you undergo a dangerous invasive procedure as a result of a faulty test result. A former editor of the American Medical Association's own journal has estimated that more than half of the tens of millions of medical tests performed yearly "do not really contribute to a patient's diagnosis or therapy." And the Centers for Disease Control have found that as much as 50 percent of simple blood and urine chemistry tests done in the top 10 percent of the laboratories in the U.S. are inaccurate. All lab test results can be expected to be incorrect a certain percentage of the time, so even the healthiest person will have an abnormal test result from time to time.

There's also the issue of defensive medicine. If the term is new to you, it is doctor-speak meaning "I gotta do the test because if I don't the litigious patient might later sue me if something goes wrong." Physicians are subjecting unsuspecting (and usually litigiously low-risk) customers to a battery of worthless pokes and probes that would send Hippocrates, if he were alive today, back to his famed Oath to add a new canon (after "First, do no harm"), which would state "Second, do no unnecessary test."

What can you do? Ensure that you have tests only when necessary and retest when appropriate. Here's how you do it:

89.

Avoid hospital laboratories and laboratories and imaging centers owned by doctors.

Hospital labs are no more reliable than independent laboratories, and they are usually considerably more expensive because the hospital overhead (cost of building, equipment, utilities) is higher.

Also, don't use a laboratory or imaging center that is owned by the physician making the referral. It just stands to reason. No judge should preside over a case in which she has a personal, vested interest. So why then let physicians refer patients to X-ray labs, specialty clinics, private hospitals, kidney dialysis units, and physical therapy practices that these same physicians either own or have a financial interest in?

In medicine it's called referral for profit, although more hard-nosed critics have labeled it a kickback scheme. The latest evidence is that doctors who have a financial interest in laboratories order four times the number of diagnostic tests as physicians with no financial investment. And a General Accounting Office study found that physician-owners of Maryland labs or imaging centers ordered, on average, 14 percent more expensive lab tests and 82 percent more expensive imaging tests than nonowner doctors.

How prevalent are these joint ventures, these investments in health care facilities by physicians in positions to refer patients for tests or services? An important Florida study, released in August 1991, found that at least 40 percent of the doctors practicing in that state have invested in joint ventures to which they can refer patients. So be on guard against the doctor more interested in protecting his investment than in healing the sick.

90.

Don't let the laboratory run more tests than you need.

You will notice that lab forms, particularly for blood and urine tests, list a number of different tests on one slip. Make sure that you and your doctor clearly indicate the specific tests that you need. Otherwise, the lab may run all the tests on the lab slip and you will be charged for them.

Routine presurgical lab tests are another problem area. They account for $30 billion a year in business, yet researchers have found that nearly half the time the tests duplicate those that patients had within the previous year. The findings indicate that normal results taken up to four months prior to surgery can be substituted safely for preoperative screening tests.

91.
If your doctor recommends an invasive procedure as the result of a laboratory test, request a retest before agreeing to the procedure.

Because of the large numbers of errors made in laboratory tests, it makes sense both financially and for the sake of your health to pay the small fee for another lab test. Erroneous lab results can expose you to expensive, dangerous, and potentially life-threatening invasive procedures. If your insurance plan requires approval for any retesting, just remind the powers-that-be that a $25 or $35 retest can save thousands in future expenses, not to mention out-of-pocket costs that are your responsibility.

92.
Investigate the use of home tests rather than laboratory tests.

Consumers are doing more to keep the doctor away, or at bay, than just eating an apple a day. Sales of do-it-yourself medical tests a few years ago topped the $500-million-a-year mark, and the best predictions have sales climbing to $1.4 billion in 1992. Sold in drugstores, in supermarkets, and through catalogs, home tests make it possible for you to take your own blood pressure, check yourself for a urinary tract infection, determine whether you're pregnant, screen yourself for certain cancers, monitor your blood sugar levels, and even predict when you're ovulating. Home testing offers a low-cost, convenient alternative to the doctor's office or lab, at least in the early stages of diagnosis.

But aside from the cost-containment angle, such testing is a good idea because it enables the consumer to involve herself in self-care and in aspects of health care once exclusively the doctor's domain. Do-it-yourself tests, however, are not without potential problems—accuracy, for one, and the situation in which your doctor just repeats the test you took at home. Most experts agree that the objective of home medical tests is for you to *work together* with your health professional to ensure the best health for yourself. Your pharmacist is a good source of information on home medical tests and can tell you what is presently available.

Remember too that not all home testing requires a kit. According to the American Cancer Society, every woman over 20 should examine her breasts monthly. Also, the most common type of cancer in humans, skin cancer, is largely curable if caught early, and you don't need a kit to check your skin for moles and suspicious and rapid changes in them.

93.

Take advantage of free testing programs at community health fairs.

Usually sponsored by hospitals and featuring a lot of giveaways along the lines of refrigerator magnets and such, health fairs offer simple screening tests: blood pressure, cholesterol, and tuberculosis screening; blood typing; vision testing, and on and on. Since these screenings are usually free, the greatest cost advantage is that you avoid having to pay for a doctor's visit unless one of the test results indicates that you need a doctor's care.

Most health fairs are set up for the purpose of getting the consumer to use (translate: buy) the services of the participating facilities or physicians. In the words of a top medical marketer, writing in *Medical Economics,* "Doctors looking for an inexpensive way to attract more patients frequently sign up with health fairs . . . just the kind of low-key marketing that many physicians like best." In other words, keep a cautious attitude, and make sure the fair promoters are providing a community service—not just an opportunity for doctors and hospitals to make a quick buck (or several hundred and more) off you.

CHAPTER 5

Insurance

Everyone hopes to stay healthy—but since there's a good chance you or a member of your family will get sick at some point, it's smart to know how to shop for the best health insurance for your money.

Most people carry health insurance, if they can afford it, or have it provided as a benefit of employment. Lately, though, you've probably noticed that your coverage is not as extensive as it once was and you're paying more in out-of-pocket expenses for deductibles and copayments. Some employers, who once provided cost-free health insurance, now require employees to make premium contributions.

For some time now, business interests have contended that their cost to provide health insurance has been increasing at a rate of 14 percent or more per year, which they say they can no longer tolerate. As a result, some companies have purchased health insurance plans that pay fewer benefits. This leaves you, the employee, facing larger and larger out-of-pocket expenses. The goal then is to maximize your health insurance benefits and reduce your out-of-pocket expense as much as possible. Here's how:

94.
Don't duplicate coverage.

Chances are you will not be permitted to collect full benefits from both policies. The insurance companies invoke a policy they call coordination of benefits, which means they compare notes to determine who owes what. They split the bill, or at least the portion that is their responsibility, and you still must pick up any copayment or deductible. In essence then, the premium for the second policy is down the drain.

95.
Don't buy disease-specific or accident insurance.

Disease-specific insurance usually covers one disease—for example, cancer or heart disease—and not only pays limited benefits but may duplicate what you already have or are about to purchase. Very limited in coverage (and for this reason not the best insurance for your money), accident insurance excludes illness but does cover medical expenses resulting from an accident. And most insurers will not allow you to collect from more than one policy for a single injury.

96.
Shop carefully for long-term-care insurance.

This insurance is also known as nursing home insurance. The most important point to ask is whether benefits are paid for any level of care: skilled, intermediate, or custodial. It's important to make sure the policy you buy pays for all three levels. Early on, long-term-care insurance paid benefits only for skilled nursing care, but today policies usually cover the full range of services available. The benefits are paid when such services are deemed medically necessary.

97.
Take advantage of the "free look" period.

After you have signed the application and paid the premium, your state may permit you to review the policy for a certain number of days—most allow 10 to 15 days—before you decide whether or not to keep it. If you are not satisfied and decide not to keep the policy, return it to the company within the time allotted and request a full refund of any premium. Call your state insurance department if you have any questions about your policy or about your state's "free look" regulation.

98.

Ask if your employer pays bounty for erroneous medical bills.

The first question a savvy medical consumer asks is "How good are my chances of finding errors?" Equifax Services, an Atlanta firm that audits around 40,000 hospital bills annually for insurers, found in one audit of selected bills that more than 97 percent of hospital bills contain errors. When the *Philadelphia Daily News* took a look at billing–again, hospital bills, in particular–in that city, it found case after case of erroneous charges. In one case, a man had his $25,185 bill for a two-week hospital stay reduced by more than $2,000 after an auditor discovered overcharges.

Many companies will pay a reward, or "bounty," to an employee who finds inaccuracies in her hospital bill that result in savings to the company. And, as you can imagine, it shouldn't be too difficult to find an error; national studies indicate that upwards of 90 percent of all hospital bills contain errors–usually in the hospital's favor. Your vigilance not only helps reduce your copayment, but your employer also benefits from the overall reduction in health insurance costs.

Don't be surprised if your insurer is not overly enthusiastic when you call to report a hospital's or doctor's overcharge. Not every company pays a reward–or even pays attention–to such diligence on your part. Insurance companies often find it easier to pay erroneous claims rather than go to the trouble of auditing the bill and possibly demanding a refund. But you and everyone else pay for overcharges, so be persistent. Be prepared to fight with your insurer over an error in your bill.

99.

Get preapproval to make sure services are covered.

Many insurance companies encourage preapproval for any procedure your doctor recommends. This just means that you submit a request to your insurance company, who will then either approve or disapprove coverage for the recommended procedure. The process of preapproval becomes even more important when there are penalties attached to bypassing the system. You may opt to have a procedure or treatment done without approval only to learn that your coverage has been reduced by half. Remember, no matter how insistent your doctor is, always check with your insurance carrier prior to any service.

100.

Pay premiums annually if you can afford to.

You may be able to receive a discount on your premium if you can pay yearly in one lump sum, or even on a semiannual basis. If you don't have an insurance plan where you work, consider asking your employer to pick up part of the premium. This way you can make the yearly premium payment and obtain a small benefit from your employment. It also saves your employer the full cost of starting a medical benefits plan.

101.

Check out local HMOs and PPOs—they may be cheaper than health insurance and offer better benefits.

Health maintenance organizations (HMOs) and preferred provider organizations (PPOs) are forms of health insurance policies as well as providers. Managed-care plans, as they are often called, are sometimes referred to as alternative delivery systems, which simply means alternatives to the traditional fee-for-service system. For the savvy medical consumer, the time to learn the rudiments of managed-care plans is *now*—as the popularity of these plans increases every year and more employers drop traditional insurance entirely and offer managed-care plans or nothing.

Health maintenance organizations come in a variety of forms, but with some elements in common:

▶ HMO members (usually called subscribers) receive comprehensive medical care for a fixed (or prepaid, meaning paid before you receive the services) monthly premium.

▶ The services are provided by an organized group of medical professionals who receive a fixed monthly payment per subscriber, regardless of the services rendered (or not rendered, whatever the case may be).

▶ Subscribers, for the most part, are limited to those physicians, hospitals, and other medical providers approved by the HMO.

A preferred provider organization, or PPO, is a group of physicians and hospitals that contract with insurance companies, unions, or employers to provide health care at negotiated fees. In return, the "preferred" group is guaranteed a volume of patients.

You need to find out when the HMOs in your area have open enrollment periods, and whether or not you meet the enrollment criteria. Also speak to your employer about offering an HMO as an option to traditional health insurance – if your company does not already. If your company offers a PPO, be aware that by joining it you will be severely limited in the providers you may use.

Consider what it would mean to you to change doctors or use a hospital that is not your favorite, should these be limitations set by the HMO or PPO. In either case, compare rates and coverage. HMOs and PPOs may (or may not) be cheaper.

102.
Use only providers who accept your insurance plan.

Some health insurers have arrangements with certain doctors and hospitals – called "participating" providers. Your policy will reimburse at a higher level if you use a participating provider.

103.

See if you're eligible for group insurance through organizations or associations to which you belong.

If you are unemployed or otherwise without an employer-subsidized health insurance policy, you may be able to obtain a less expensive group policy through organizations or associations to which you belong—and you may not have to look any further than your mailbox. Many fraternal, alumni, and civic associations have health insurance plans for sale. While many of these offerings are indemnity plans—i.e., they pay a fixed amount per day in the hospital or per service—in a pinch they can cover at least some of your expenses.

Some states are now offering low-cost insurance for disabled and/or handicapped persons who are unable to obtain private insurance. Contact your state insurance department or department of welfare to see if it is available where you live and if you are eligible.

104.

Donate blood—join a blood bank.

By committing yourself to the donation of a specified amount of blood per year, you can receive insurance coverage for blood supplies for yourself and possibly for your family as well.

105.

Join an ambulance service.

Just as with a blood bank, private and voluntary ambulance services will often offer a specified amount of service for a yearly donation.

106.

Check all employer-sponsored health insurance plan options carefully.

A happy scenario is one where your employer, as many larger companies are doing, offers a wide range of policies and options at varying costs. Many workers are offered a "cafeteria package" of benefits and must choose from an assortment of possibilities. Unfortunately, too many people decide by the toss of a coin–an uninformed and hardly savvy decision-making tactic. To get the best value for your money, carefully compare all the policies with *your needs* in mind. Do not settle for less coverage than you need. Your premium for more coverage may not be much higher.

107.

Pay premiums on time.

An insurance company can cancel your policy if you fail to pay the premiums or continually pay the premiums late. Be sure to keep on top of any necessary employee deductions if yours is an employer-sponsored policy.

108.

Know what your state insurance department can do for you in the way of consumer protection.

Your state insurance department plays an important role in regulating insurance companies. Beyond licensing insurance companies and agents, approving policies that are sold, and mandating minimum benefits for policies–the department has the power to conduct investigations, take testimony, hold hearings, and render verdicts. As such, your state insurance department may also be able to help you if you have a problem with an insurance company or agent. Any formal complaint you file with the department will be investigated and, if possible, resolved.

HOW TO FILE A COMPLAINT
WITH YOUR STATE INSURANCE DEPARTMENT

Your complaint should be in writing and contain the following information:

- ► Your name, address, and telephone number.
- ► The name, address, and telephone number of your insurance company.
- ► The identification number of your policy.
- ► The type of policy.
- ► The nature of your complaint: the premium, the coverage, a claim, or the actions of your agent.

Make sure you keep copies of everything you send to the department. You must be willing to follow through on your complaint and appear at any hearings if so directed. If the law and the facts are on your side, the insurance department can usually help resolve the problem.

CHAPTER 6

Nursing Home and Home Health Care

The term "nursing home" is actually a very general name for several different types of medical care facilities. It has the connotation of being a "last stop" for the elderly, but it can actually be a place for people of all ages to convalesce following an accident or serious illness, or a temporary placement for an older person while the family shops around and lines up alternative modes of care. A common classification for nursing homes is the level of care they provide:

▶ *Skilled nursing.* Care is delivered by registered and licensed practical nurses on the orders of an attending physician. The person who requires skilled nursing is often bedridden and not able to help himself or herself.

▶ *Intermediate care.* The intermediate care facility provides less intensive care than the skilled facility and usually costs less; the care there stresses rehabilitation therapy to enable the resident to go home or at least regain or retain as many functions of daily living as possible. Care is delivered by registered and licensed practical nurses and an array of therapists.

▶ *Sheltered, or custodial, care.* This level of care is nonmedical in that residents do not require constant attention from nurses or aides, but do need help with such routine activities as getting out of bed, walking, eating, and bathing.

One in every five people can expect to need extended nursing care at some time in their lives. To make matters worse, very few basic health insurance policies cover nursing home care for more than a few days or weeks. Even Medicare, the federal health insurance plan for senior citizens, does not cover what we think of as long-term care. Medicare covers a limited number of days of skilled nursing facility care only, and is primarily intended to permit recovery outside of a hospital. So if you or a member of your family needs such care, you must know how to get quality care without paying more than necessary.

What follows are ways for the savvy medical consumer to get the best value in extended nursing care. Knowing all of your options is the key.

109.

Check the yellow pages for the visiting nurse association and other agencies that provide home health care.

The first thing to know is that nursing home placement is not, and should not be, the sole solution to the plight of an older person who is debilitated by ill health and who has increasing difficulty taking care of himself or herself. Nothing mandates nursing home placement if there is someone available to administer the needed care in the home or to coordinate delivery of alternative services. Visiting nurse associations (VNAs) are the oldest home health care agencies in most communities; however, they aren't the only agencies that provide home health services. Hospitals, not-for-profit community organizations, and for-profit agencies are also in the home care business. VNAs provide referrals to other community services when appropriate.

Familiarize yourself with the various levels of care available in your community. Full-service agencies, such as the VNA and certified home health agencies, offer everything from skilled nursing care to homemaker services. If you're responsible for the full cost of the services, don't contract for more care than you need. Another important point to consider is whether or not the agency is certified. This could become rather important if your health insurance plan will cover only services from a certified agency. These groups can provide you with information on certified home care agencies:

National League for Nursing
350 Hudson Street
New York, NY 10014
212-989-9393

Joint Commission on the Accreditation of
    Healthcare Organizations
One Renaissance Boulevard
Oakbrook, IL 60181
708-916-5600

National HomeCaring Council
519 C Street, N.E.
Washington, DC 20002
202-547-6586

For information on home health services, contact:

Foundation for Hospice and Home Care
519 C Street, N.E.
Washington, DC 20002
202-547-6586

National Association for Home Care
519 C Street, N.E.
Washington, DC 20002
202-547-7424

110.
Use adult day care.

An adult day care center lets an elderly person enjoy a full range
of activities – including arts and crafts, games, and just plain old
conversation – on a daily basis in a supervised setting. Communities nationwide are establishing such facilities, which provide a
degree of supervision and appropriate activities for elderly persons
with minor physical disabilities but do not provide nursing care.

It is well established that elderly people remain healthier if
they are able to continue to live in their own homes – and it's
usually cheaper, too. Adult day care can often make the
difference between being able to remain at home and needing
institutionalization.

111.

Use home health care.

Home health agencies can provide services ranging from help with cooking and cleaning to full nursing care at home. For the elderly person with minor disabilities, a person to cook or clean is often all the support that's needed. A home health agency can help you evaluate the help that you need. But don't purchase any more care than necessary.

Bear in mind too that home health care is not just for the elderly on Medicare. Many people under age 65, who are not yet legally disabled–and who therefore would not normally qualify for Medicare–but who require rehabilitative or chronic care, are eligible to use home care programs. Home health services offer an opportunity for early discharge from a hospital or a skilled nursing facility, and in fact such specialized or rehabilitation services often meet a person's long-term needs more efficiently than acute care hospital settings.

If you are eligible for Medicare, know the limits of coverage of home health care. If you are not on Medicare, find out what your insurance plan pays and what eligibility requirements you must meet. Generally, a doctor must arrange for such services as part-time home nursing care, occupational therapy, speech therapy, and special meals and other nutritional services to be furnished in your home.

112.

If you need nursing home care, purchase the lowest level necessary.

Of the three levels of nursing home care–skilled, intermediate, and custodial–skilled care is the most expensive because care is provided by registered and licensed practical nurses on the orders of an attending physician. Remember, skilled care is the only level of care that Medicare will reimburse for, and then only a very limited amount of coverage is provided.

For information on nursing home care, contact:

American Health Care Association
1201 L Street, N.W.
Washington, DC 20005
202-842-4444

American Association of Homes for the Aging
901 E Street, N.W., Suite 500
Washington, DC 20004
202-783-2242

National Consumers League
815 15th Street, N.W., Suite 928
Washington, DC 20005
202-639-8140

QUICK CHECKLIST OF QUESTIONS FOR NURSING HOME ADMINISTRATORS

Even before you spend your time going around to various nursing homes, touring them, and interviewing administrators, you should conduct phone interviews to establish a base of information on which to build. Find out:

1. What level of care is offered?
2. Are there special restrictions on the types of patients accepted?
3. How many beds (for the type of care you need) does the home provide?
4. Is there a waiting list, and if so, approximately how long is it?
5. What type of license or accreditation does the home have?
6. Does the home accept Medicare and Medicaid?
7. Is there an initial deposit required, and, if so, how much is it?
8. What are the monthly room charges?
9. Are additional monthly services provided? What are their charges?

113.

Use Meals on Wheels and/or other programs that are alternatives to institutionalization.

An excellent program designed to provide hot, nutritious meals to homebound older people, Meals on Wheels is usually operated by a social service agency or community group. The service delivers one hot meal a day directly to the person's residence, and the price of such a service is nominal, often based on ability to pay.

As with a number of other programs for those people who do not require constant supervision or that much nursing care, Meals on Wheels may actually delay a person's need for a nursing home for many years. The savvy medical consumer will explore the other programs as well: *homemaker services*, for people who require some assistance in the preparation of meals or with housework; *home sharing*, an arrangement in which a resident manager and a few older people share housing and share expenses; *telephone reassurance*, a formal or informal system to take away the risk of total isolation for the elderly person living alone; *shopping services*, which entail having groceries and other needed items delivered; *special transportation services*, consisting of vehicles equipped to handle wheelchairs and other devices, for people with limited mobility; and *special health aids or devices*, such as walkers, mechanical feeding devices, geriatric chairs, and artificial limbs, which can facilitate personal independence or make it more feasible for a family member to assist. Contact your local, county, or state welfare or human services agencies for availability of or more information about these programs.

114.

Use a hospice.

Hospices are for people who are terminally ill, and their mission is to inspirit death with dignity and allow the family close contact with the patient, free from the intrusive high technology of the hospital. Less expensive than a hospital because they do not use life-sustaining technologies, a hospice provides basic medical care, counseling for the patient and family, and prescribed pain relievers. Most hospices will care for patients for whom a doctor's prognosis indicates that they have fewer than six months to live. Some hospices come to a person's home and provide services, while others actually operate a facility where the patient resides. For information on hospice care, contact:

>Children's Hospice International
>901 N. Washington Street, Suite 700
>Alexandria, VA 22314
>800-242-4453

>Hospice Education Institute
>5 Essex Square, Suite 3-B
>Essex, CT 06426
>800-331-1620

>National Hospice Organization
>1901 North Moore Street, Suite 901
>Alexandria, VA 22209
>800-658-8898

115.
Investigate life care communities.

A relatively new concept, these communities provide residential care in an apartment-like setting, along with skilled and intermediate nursing care. As residents require nursing care, they are transferred to the nursing home section of the community, and once they recover return to their apartments. The life care community covers all costs of hospitalization, so, as you can imagine, the services do not come cheap. This option often requires a substantial, nonrefundable down payment as well as monthly fees. A good source of information on life care communities is available from:

>American Association of Homes for the Aging
>901 E Street, N.W., Suite 500
>Washington, DC 20004
>202-783-2242

116.

Prepare for the financial costs of nursing home care.

Nursing home care is expensive, costing you anywhere from
$20,000 to $35,000 per year, depending on the level of care.
Many insurance companies are now offering long-term-care
insurance–specifically designed to cover nursing home care. If
you're going to purchase such a policy, a good rule of thumb is
to select a policy that pays at least $60 per day, for a period of at
least four years. Look for a policy that will keep up with inflation.
A present benefit of $60 a day could easily dwindle to a future
value of only $20 due to inflation. To obtain a list of insurance
companies offering long-term-care policies, contact:

> Health Insurance Association of America
> P. O. Box 41455
> Washington, DC 20018

Also look into your eligibility for Medicaid. Medicaid is the
government health insurance program that will pay for nursing
home care when most of a person's assets have been depleted.
The fact is that most people in nursing homes for any length of
time usually end up using the Medicaid program.

CHAPTER 7

Medical Equipment

Durable medical equipment such as hospital beds and wheelchairs can be extremely valuable tools in caring for an ill person at home–*and* can save you money in the process. Anything that enables a sick person to remain at home rather than in an institution makes dollars and sense.

Now the bad news. According to recent government reports, some unethical medical equipment companies have targeted Medicare beneficiaries as easy marks for purchasing medical equipment. The scam usually starts with a letter or telephone call to beneficiaries telling them that they are eligible for a particular piece of medical equipment and that Medicare will pay for it. The problem here is that the equipment may or may not be needed, and if it isn't medically necessary Medicare will not pay for it. And guess who gets stuck with the bill?

If you know what to look for and what to do, you can save money on durable medical equipment. Here are our suggestions:

117.
Borrow medical equipment whenever possible.

Most home health aids can be borrowed from various community organizations. Ask your local home health organization or visiting nurse association. If no such services are available in your area, you may be able to rent the required equipment from a local pharmacy. But before renting, check to see if your insurance policy will cover its purchase. Also shop around; rental prices for equipment vary from dealer to dealer. If you need the equipment for a long period of time, you will probably have to purchase it.

118.
Save by owning medical self-care equipment.

Simple self-care equipment such as thermometers, blood pressure cuffs, stethoscopes, and otoscopes are helpful devices, especially when it comes to making informed choices concerning your need for doctor's help. Many are available from discount mail-order companies. Check out a number of suppliers to find a high quality item at a reasonable price.

119.
Check out the equipment's reliability before purchasing.

Every piece of equipment you purchase should come with literature that describes its reliability within a certain range. For instance, thermometers may be reliable within a range of one degree Fahrenheit. Some equipment will be more reliable than others. The equipment's accompanying literature should also describe the period of time the equipment can be expected to maintain this degree of reliability without servicing.

120.
Find out where servicing is available.

Equipment such as blood pressure cuffs must be periodically serviced to maintain reliability. Make sure that you know how, where, and how often a piece of equipment must be serviced before you purchase it. In fact, it makes sense to purchase only equipment with a written warranty. Further, you will save money if the equipment you buy can be serviced locally.

121.

Check the supplier with the Better Business Bureau, and with Medicare if the equipment is for a Medicare beneficiary.

For many health items such as hearing aids, it is wise to see if your local Better Business Bureau has any complaints on file against the supplier from whom you are thinking of purchasing. If the equipment is prescribed for a Medicare beneficiary, determine if the supplier is a certified Medicare supplier. What this means is that the supplier will accept the Medicare-approved amount as payment in full and will bill the beneficiary only for the 20 percent copayment.

122.

Check for sales.

With health and medical equipment, just as with most other consumer items, suppliers often offer sales. Purchasing items on sale is always a good way to save money.

123.

Return any medical equipment that arrives unsolicited.

Some doctors and medical suppliers target Medicare beneficiaries with offers of so-called free equipment paid for by Medicare. In addition, some equipment manufacturers use well-known personalities to hawk various products ranging from special beds to power-assisted chairs. Be aware that Medicare will pay only for durable medical equipment that's ordered by your doctor, as long as it is medically necessary. The words "medically necessary" are the key here. Unless your doctor specifically orders equipment, do not respond to any mail order or telephone marketing schemes.

CHAPTER 8

Prevention

Preventive measures have the potential to save you more money on health costs than anything else you do. Even more important, prevention is health promotion, something every savvy medical consumer should be doing more of. But the bad news is that—as 58 cents out of every health care dollar go to doctors and hospitals—only two cents go to health promotion activities. That's all we spend to keep ourselves healthy.

However, you have many opportunities in daily living to get your two cents' worth by doing things to improve your health. Remember, the sooner you start, the healthier you will be.

124.
Learn stress-reduction techniques.

There are techniques—some simple, others requiring professional help—that can help you lower your stress level. Strong evidence exists that those under stress, or those who cope poorly with stress, are less healthy than others. And at the very least that adds up to a lot of extra dollars spent on medical care.

125.
Quit smoking.

Smoking increases a person's risk for a number of major diseases: heart disease, stroke, and cancer. But beyond that, smokers are just generally more prone to illness—and therefore lose more work time due to illness—than nonsmokers. If you are a smoker, consider also the increased risk at which you put your friends and family as they breathe in your exhaled smoke. Save money and your health by throwing away your cigarettes.

126.
Don't do anything to excess.

Old wisdom, but true today. Excessive eating, drinking, smoking, and even exercise can be harmful and expensive.

127.
Make your home injury-proof.

Inspect your home for safety. Check electrical cords, the condition of carpeting, the placement of furniture, and so on. Additions such as nonslip strips on bathtubs are inexpensive ways to ensure your safety and prevent the need for costly medical care.

128.
Maintain desirable weight.

This does not necessarily mean that you should weigh what those famous charts say you should weigh, but you will be healthier if you weigh what feels good for you. And you'll save money on health care as well.

129.
Wear seat belts.

Many new cars employ a passive-restraint system that auto-matically fastens your seat belt; however, you may still need to manually fasten the lap belt. Whatever the case, you're always safer when you use the safety equipment that is included with your car. Fifty thousand deaths a year, untold pain and suffering, and loss of income should be enough to convince anyone to use seat belts.

130.

Always properly restrain children in cars.

Remember—*you* are responsible for the safety of your children. It's a good idea to take along a car seat on airplanes and other forms of transportation, too. Injury prevention saves money and incalculable suffering.

131.

Avoid processed foods.

Processed foods usually contain more fat, more salt, and less fiber than unprocessed foods. They also contain preservatives and other chemicals. The healthier you are, the more money you will save on costly medical care—so pass the bran.

132.

Have microwave emissions checked.

Call the authorized repair service recommended in the literature accompanying your microwave. (Indeed, your manual should include a maintenance schedule.) A repair service should be able to do a quick, low-cost emission check. Microwave emissions are potentially harmful, so a few dollars for a check can save you medical costs in the future.

133.

Purchase basic medical tools for self-diagnosis.

You can save yourself time and expense by having basic medical tools such as a blood pressure cuff (sphygmomanometer), an otoscope (for looking in the ears), and a stethoscope. Used in combination with a good medical guide, you can avoid many unnecessary visits to the doctor.

134.
Join the People's Medical Society.

The People's Medical Society *Newsletter* and our many other publications offer you an easy-to-read supply of medical information that you can use to make informed decisions about your health care.

135.
Plan a fire escape route, and hold home fire drills.

Simple fire-safety measures such as smoke alarms—an ample number placed strategically in your home—and fire drills can prevent serious injury or worse in the event of a home fire.

136.
Exercise regularly.

Regular exercise protects against heart disease, osteoporosis, and a variety of other common illnesses. It will also help you maintain a desirable weight. Joining a health club is cheaper than health care for a chronic illness such as heart disease.

137.
Make friends, and purchase a pet.

Studies have shown that people who are socially active are healthier than those who are "loners." Check your local newspaper for singles activities at churches, social organizations, Parents Without Partners, exercise clubs, and so on. Place an ad in the personals section of newspapers and magazines, or be daring and answer one!

Pets make great companions, and there are many dogs and cats at your local animal shelter just waiting for adoption. You'll have a lifelong friend and the satisfaction that comes with helping a less fortunate creature. How you feel mentally has long been connected to how you feel physically, and being socially active or having a pet are two ways to improve your health. And remember, the cost for dog and cat food is considerably less than the cost of multiple doctor visits and prescription medications.

138.
Wear a lead apron for dental X rays.

You should always shield the parts of your body not being X-rayed. Excessive radiation is a definite health hazard—and why invite trouble (and additional costs) when there's a simple remedy?

139.
Keep current with immunizations.

Adults need to be reimmunized periodically for tetanus and, in some areas of the country, other diseases as well. These immunizations often are given free or at a very low cost through community groups. Elderly adults, in particular, should consider immunization against influenza and pneumonia.

140.
Avoid too much exposure to the sun.

Dermatologists have definitely identified a link between exposure to the sun and skin cancer; however, you don't have to live in a cave. Some commonsense approaches to the sun are: Always use a sunscreen with a sun protection factor (SPF) of 15 or more; keep your exposure to a minimum; don't get all your sun at once; and wear protective clothing such as a hat or long-sleeved shirt when in the sun.

For more information on how to enjoy the sun and avoid the hazards, contact:

Skin Cancer Foundation
475 Park Avenue
New York, NY 10016

141.
Wash your hands.

Frequent hand washing will lower your chances of catching colds, flu, and other contagious diseases.

142.
Take a vacation.

Everyone needs and benefits from periodic breaks in the daily routine. Listen to yourself–don't get too "burned out" before you give yourself a break. Hotels are cheaper than hospitals.

143.
Get enough sleep.

Most people need seven to eight hours of sleep per day. Again, listen to yourself and make sure you get what you need.

144.
Eat lots of fiber.

Increasing the amount of fiber in your diet is the easiest way to lower your risk of colon cancer. It will also help with constipation. Laxatives are much more expensive than an extra piece of whole wheat bread.

145.
Drink cranberry juice.

Cranberry juice can be protective against bladder infections. But be careful to avoid the juices with added sugar and corn syrups. Cranberry juice is cheaper than antibiotics–and a lot more fun to ingest.

146.

Brush your teeth and floss daily.

Good oral hygiene is essential to good general health, so don't forget to brush and floss your teeth on a daily basis. Failure to develop and practice good oral health habits can be counter-productive to all your efforts at staying healthy. In addition, one unforeseen dental bill can wipe out any savings you've accumulated by practicing good general health.

Buy a plaque removal system for you and your family. Gum disease is one of the leading causes of tooth loss, and the cost to replace lost teeth can be quite high.

147.

Contact a self-help support group.

For many illnesses, a self-help support group can be as helpful as your doctor in speeding your recovery. Self-help support groups are in the business of empowerment, giving consumers the information and strategies they need to successfully deal with their conditions. In addition, in such groups you meet people who share your condition and with whom you can share a common bond. For more information on self-help groups, contact:

American Self-Help Clearinghouse
St. Clares-Riverside Medical Center
Denville, NJ 07834
201-625-7101

National Self-Help Clearinghouse
City University of New York
Graduate Center, Room 620
25 West 43rd Street
New York, NY 10036
212-642-2944

148.

Practice safe sex.

Unfortunately and undeniably, sexually transmitted diseases—gonorrhea, herpes, syphilis, acquired immunodeficiency syndrome (AIDS), just to name a few—are a nasty fact of life. Most at risk are those people who have many sexual partners. The risks, however, are minimized if a condom is always used during intercourse.

149.

Know the number for your local poison control center.

Calling for help immediately if you suspect someone in your family has ingested a poisonous substance can make the difference between a minor digestive disturbance and a week in the hospital's intensive care unit. Prompt action saves lives and money.

150.

Wear appropriate protective clothing when playing sports or engaging in recreational activities.

Whether the activity is bicycling or football, protective clothing can spare participants from easily preventable injuries. Preventing injuries or lessening their severity saves money.

Adverse reaction: Reaction that harms a person in some way.

Advocate: Person who represents another's interests.

Antihistamine: Medication used to treat allergies and cold symptoms such as itchy eyes and a runny nose.

Assignment: Process by which a doctor or hospital agrees to file an insurance claim in exchange for direct payment from the insurer. Under the Medicare system, the physician or hospital must also agree to accept that direct payment, plus any required patient copayments, as payment in full.

Audiologist: Medical practitioner (non-M.D.) who specializes in treating hearing problems.

Board certification: Medical specialty boards, such as the American College of Obstetricians and Gynecologists and the American Academy of Family Physicians, certify physicians in their respective specialties through a process of testing and evaluating qualifications.

Cesarean section: Method of delivering a baby by abdominal surgery.

Chiropractor: Medical practitioner (D.C.) who focuses on improving nerve function through manipulation and adjustment of body parts, particularly the spine.

Consultation: Discussion between physicians about a medical case or its treatment, for which the patient is billed.

Contraindication: Something that makes a particular medication or treatment inadvisable.

Copayment: Payment required of the patient in addition to the payment made by the insurance company. A copayment may be in the form of a deductible or a percentage payment (for instance, the insurance company pays 80 percent and the patient pays 20 percent).

Custodial care: Provision of room, board, and personal services, generally on a long-term basis, without additional medical services.

Decongestant: Medication that acts to clear congestion. It helps such symptoms as stuffy nose or chest congestion.

Deductible: Amount a patient is required to pay before his or her insurance company will begin to make payments.

Diagnosis: Identification of a patient's illness through consideration of the signs and symptoms.

Drug: Substance other than food that is intended to influence the functions of the body.

Family practitioner: Medical practitioner who specializes in treating the whole family, from uncomplicated births to care of the elderly.

For-profit: A business that operates to make more money than it requires to continue operating.

Generic drug: Drug that is a copy of a brand name drug.

Group insurance coverage: Insurance policy that covers a group of people. Such insurance is generally cheaper than individual coverage because the insurance risks are spread out among the group.

Health maintenance organization (HMO): Organization of medical providers that contracts with patients to offer specific services in exchange for a prepaid premium.

Hospice: Organization that provides specialized care for dying patients either in their home or at a facility.

Intermediate care facility: Facility that provides less intensive care than a skilled nursing facility. Patients are generally more mobile, and rehabilitation therapies are stressed.

Invasive treatment: Medical treatment that involves the invasion of the body with a drug or an instrument.

Itemized bill: Bill that lists each item and service and its corresponding charge.

Living will: Document that indicates a person's treatment wishes in the event that he or she is unable to verbally communicate those wishes. A living will is usually used as written authorization for the non-use or removal of life-sustaining treatments.

Midwife: Medical practitioner, often a nurse, who specializes in caring for women and delivering babies.

Nonprofit: Organization that functions by earning just enough money to continue operating.

Nosocomial infection: Infection acquired in the hospital.

Nurse practitioner: Nurse who has received specialized training that enables him or her to provide basic diagnostic medical care to patients.

Optometrist: Medical practitioner (O.D.) who specializes in examining eyes and who is able to prescribe corrective lenses but not perform surgery or invasive treatments.

Over-the-counter (OTC) drug: Drug that is available without a doctor's prescription.

Physician's assistant: Medical practitioner who is specially trained to provide a basic level of diagnostic medical care, usually under the supervision of a physician.

Physician's Desk Reference (PDR): A comprehensive reference book primarily listing prescription drugs and indications for use, contraindications, and dosages.

Podiatrist: Medical practitioner (D.P.M.) who specializes in caring for feet.

Preferred provider organization (PPO): Similar to an HMO, an organization of health care providers that contracts with patients for a specific amount of service in exchange for a prepaid premium.

Prescription drug: Drug that can be purchased only with a doctor's prescription.

Second opinion: An objective evaluation, diagnosis, and treatment recommendation from a medical practitioner concerning a health problem that has previously been evaluated by another medical practitioner.

Side effect: Effect of a drug or treatment that is not directly a part of the healing process.

Skilled nursing facility (SNF): An institution that offers nursing services similar to those given in a hospital, to aid recuperation of those who are seriously ill.